歯科衛生学シリーズ

歯科英語

一般社団法人
全国歯科衛生士教育協議会　監修

医歯薬出版株式会社

＜執筆者一覧＞

●執筆者（*執筆者代表）

Thomas R. Ward*　大阪歯科大学非常勤講師
川口　陽子　東京医科歯科大学名誉教授
廣瀬　浩二　東京農業大学農学部外国語研究室教授
杉田めぐみ　神田外語大学外国語学部准教授

●編　集

矢尾　和彦　元大阪歯科大学歯科衛生士専門学校校長
高阪　利美　愛知学院大学特任教授
合場千佳子　日本歯科大学東京短期大学教授

This book is originally published in Japanese
under the title of :
SHIKAEISEIGAKU－SHIRĪZU
SHIKAEIGO
(The Science of Dental Hygiene：A Series of Textbooks — Dental English)
Edited by The Japan Association for Dental Hygienist Education

ISHIYAKU PUBLISHERS, INC
7-10, Honkomagome 1 chome, Bunkyo-ku,
Tokyo 113-8612, Japan

『歯科衛生学シリーズ』の誕生

全国歯科衛生士教育協議会が監修を行ってきた歯科衛生士養成のための教科書のタイトルを，従来の『最新歯科衛生士教本』から『歯科衛生学シリーズ』に変更させていただくことになりました．2022 年度は新たに改訂された教科書 2 点を, 2023 年度からはすべての教科書のタイトルを『歯科衛生学シリーズ』とさせていただきます．

全衛協が監修及び編集を行ってきた教科書としては,『歯科衛生士教本』,『新歯科衛生士教本』,『最新歯科衛生士教本』があり，その時代にあわせて改訂・発刊をしてきました．しかし, これまでの『歯科衛生士教本』には「歯科衛生士」という職種名がついていたため，医療他職種からは職業としての「業務マニュアル」を彷彿させると，たびたび指摘されてきました．さらに，一部の歯科医師からは歯科衛生士の教育に学問は必要ないという誤解を生む素地にもなっていたようです．『歯科衛生学シリーズ』というタイトルには，このような指摘・誤解に応えるとともに学問としての【歯科衛生学】を示す目的もあるのです．

『歯科衛生学シリーズ』誕生の背景には，全国歯科衛生士教育協議会の 2021 年 5 月の総会で承認された「歯科衛生学の体系化」という歯科衛生士の教育および業務に関する大きな改革案の公開があります．この報告では,「口腔の健康を通して全身の健康の維持・増進をはかり，生活の質の向上に資するためのもの」を「歯科衛生」と定義し，この「歯科衛生」を理論と実践の両面から探求する学問が【歯科衛生学】であるとしました．【歯科衛生学】は基礎歯科衛生学・臨床歯科衛生学・社会歯科衛生学の 3 つの分野から構成されるとしています．また, 令和 4 年には歯科衛生士国家試験出題基準も改定されたことから, 各分野の新しい『歯科衛生学シリーズ』の教科書の編集を順次進めております．

教育年限が 3 年以上に引き上げられて，短期大学や 4 年制大学も 2 桁の数に増加し,「日本歯科衛生教育学会」など【歯科衛生学】の教育に関連する学会も設立され,【歯科衛生学】の体系化も提案された今，自分自身の知識や経験が整理され，視野の広がりは臨床上の疑問を解くための指針ともなり，自分が実践してきた歯科保健・医療・福祉の正当性を検証することも可能となります．日常の身近な問題を見つけ，科学的思考によって自ら問題を解決する能力を養い，歯科衛生業務を展開していくことが令和の時代に求められています．

2023 年 1 月

一般社団法人　全国歯科衛生士教育協議会理事長

眞木　吉信

最新歯科衛生士教本の監修にあたって

歯科衛生士教育は，昭和24年に始まり，60年近くが経過しました．この間，歯科保健に対する社会的ニーズの高まりや歯科医学・医療の発展に伴い，歯科衛生士教育にも質的・量的な充実が叫ばれ，法制上の整備や改正が行われてきました．平成17年4月からは，高齢化の進展，医療の高度化・専門化などの環境変化に伴い，引き続いて歯科衛生士の資質の向上をはかることを目的とし，修業年限が3年以上となります．

21世紀を担っていく歯科衛生士には，これまで以上にさまざまな課題が課せられております．高齢化の進展により生活習慣病を有した患者さんが多くなり，現場で活躍していくためには，手技の習得はもちろんのこと，患者さんの全身状態をよく知り口腔との関係を考慮しながら対応していく必要があります．また，一人の患者さんにはいろいろな人々が関わっており，これらの人々と連携し，患者さんにとってよりよい支援ができるような歯科衛生士としての視点と能力が求められています．そのためには，まず業務の基盤となる知識を整えることが基本となります．

全国歯科衛生士教育協議会は，こうした社会的要請に対応するべく，歯科衛生士教育の問題を研究・協議し，教育の向上と充実をはかって参りました．活動の一環として，昭和42年には多くの関係者が築いてこられた教育内容を基に「歯科衛生士教本」，平成3年には「新歯科衛生士教本」を編集いたしました．そして，今回，「最新歯科衛生士教本」を監修いたしました．本最新シリーズは，「歯科衛生士の資質向上に関する検討会」で提示された内容をふまえ，今後の社会的要請に応えられる歯科衛生士を養成するために構成，編集されております．また，全国の歯科大学や歯学部，歯科衛生士養成施設，関係諸機関で第一線で活躍されている先生方がご執筆されており，内容も歯科衛生士を目指す学生諸君ができるだけ理解しやすいよう，平易に記載するなどの配慮がなされております．

本協議会としては，今後，これからの時代の要請により誕生した教本として本最新シリーズが教育の場で十分に活用され，わが国の歯科保健の向上・発展に大いに寄与することを期待しております．

終わりに本シリーズの監修にあたり，種々のご助言とご支援をいただいた先生方，ならびに全国の歯科衛生士養成施設の関係者に，心より厚く御礼申し上げます．

2007年1月

全国歯科衛生士教育協議会　会長　櫻井善忠

発刊の辞

近年，国民の健康に対する関心が高まるとともに，高齢者や要介護者の増加によって歯科医療サービスにおける歯科衛生士の役割が大きく変化してきました．そのため，歯科衛生士は口腔の保健を担う者として，これまでにも増して広い知識と高度な技能が求められるようになり，歯科医学の進歩や社会の変化に即した教育が必要になりました．

歯科衛生士養成教育は，このような社会の要請に応じるために平成 17 年 4 月，歯科衛生士学校養成所指定規則が一部改正されて教育内容の見直しと修業年限の延長が図られ，原則として平成 22 年までにすべての養成機関が 3 年以上の教育をすることになりました．

このような状況の下に発刊された最新歯科衛生士教本シリーズでは，基礎分野の教本として生物，化学，英語，心理学をとりあげました．これらは，従来の歯科衛生士教本シリーズの中でも発刊していましたが，今回の最新シリーズの発刊にあたり，目次立てから新たに編纂しました．とくに生物と化学は，医療関係職種に共通する科学の基礎知識を系統的に学習できるように，高校の初歩レベルから専門基礎分野で学ぶ生化学，生理学などにつながる内容を網羅しています．

英語は，歯科診療室における様々な場面を想定した会話文をベースに，練習問題や単語，リーディングテキストを豊富にとりあげ，教育目標のレベルに応じて幅広い授業展開ができるように心掛けました．

また，心理学では，一般的な心理学の知識はもちろん，歯科衛生士が患者との信頼関係に基づく医療サービスを提供する能力および歯科医師や他の医療職種の人たちと円滑な人間関係を保つ能力を修得するための基盤となる内容を併せもつ教本としました．

これらの教本がテキストとしてだけでなく，卒業後も座右の書として活用されることを期待しています．

2007 年 1 月

最新歯科衛生士教本編集委員

可児　徳子　矢尾　和彦　松井　恭平　眞木　吉信

高阪　利美　合場千佳子　白鳥たかみ

執筆の序

「英語は世界の共通語」これに異を唱える人はほとんどいないでしょう．いまや英語は，イギリス，アメリカ，オーストラリアなど，それを母国語とする人たちだけのものではなく，世界中でコミュニケーションツールとして使われています．

日本に来る外国人の数は年々増えています．ビジネスや休暇で短期滞在する人もいますし，居住者として日本各地でさまざまな職業に携わる人もいます．外国人の患者さんが歯科医院を訪れる機会も珍しくはありません．そんな患者さんと意思疎通をすることは，歯科衛生士として大変重要なことです．薬の飲み方や病歴の聞き取りなど，治療に直接関わることを伝えなければいけないのはもちろんのことですが，言葉の壁に阻まれて心細い思いをしている患者さんと英語でコミュニケーションが取れれば，彼らの不安感をなくし，ひいては患者さんの信頼を得ることができます．

Part1では，受付業務，インフォームドコンセント，口腔衛生指導など，臨床でのさまざまな場面を想定した会話例を掲載しました．歯科のプロではない患者さんと話すことが目的ですから，難しい構文や専門用語などはなるべく使わず，あくまで短くて分かりやすい文章になるよう心がけました．会話は言葉のキャッチボールですからListeningを使って聞き取りの練習もできるように，またPair Workなどで基本の会話の応用練習もできるように編集しました．Readingでは口腔衛生に関する興味ある話題の読み物を載せましたので，少し難しいかもしれませんがチャレンジして読んでみてください．

Part2では，歯科に関係する単語のほか，頻出語の日英対訳，患者さんや子どもに分かりやすい表現，例文など実際に使いやすいようにまとめました．

Part3では，海外では歯科衛生士がどのような仕事をしているか，という話題を掲載しました．国内の事情と比較してみると興味深いでしょう．

この本は在学中の教科書としてだけでなく，卒業後も勉強を続けていけるように，すぐに開ける参考書として手元において活用していただきたいと思います．実際に歯科医院で外国人の患者さんと話すときのみならず，将来，学会や歯科医院の見学などで外国に行くときにも，本書が少しでも役立つことを望んでやみません．

なお，Part1の Warm up と Dialogue はThomas R. Ward，Vocabulary, Listening, Pair Workなどは杉田めぐみ，Readingは川口陽子，Part2は川口陽子，廣瀬浩二，Part3は廣瀬浩二が担当しました．本書の編纂にあたり，いろいろ貴重なご助言をくださった矢尾和彦先生をはじめ，基礎科目を統括していただいた編集委員の高阪利美先生，合場千佳子先生に心より感謝いたします．

2007年3月

Thomas R. Ward

CONTENTS

Part2 Important Vocabulary for Dental Hygienists ······ 127

Part3 歯科衛生士の仕事とは ······ 149

コラム

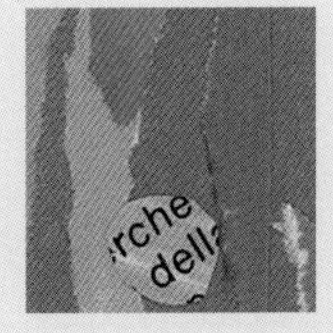

Part 1

English Conversation for Dental Hygienists

各DialogueおよびListening問題の音声ファイルについては，https://www.ishiyaku.co.jp/pickup/428330.aspxよりダウンロードして下さい（音声ファイル名は，本書の該当ページに記載しています）．各Listeningの問題文・解答についても，上記サイトにて公開しております．

1 Making an Appointment by Telephone

Warm up

When a patient calls for an appointment, the receptionist should first determine if he wants a regular examination and cleaning, or if there is a problem that needs immediate attention. Ideally, all patients should come in for their recall examination and cleaning so they will not have dental emergencies.

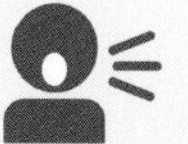

Vocabulary

appointment 〈名〉予約，約束
receptionist 〈名〉受付
examination 〈名〉検査　***cf.*** examine 〈動〉検査する，調べる
cleaning 〈名〉クリーニング（口腔清掃）
immediate 〈形〉即時の，緊急の
attention 〈名〉注意，手当て
recall 〈名〉リコール（歯科では「定期検診」の意味）
emergency 〈名〉緊急　***cf.*** emergent 〈形〉緊急の，急患の

I'm a Dental Hygienist!

263-00488

Dialogue

音声：01-D.mp3

Situation Ms. Hernandez is calling to make an appointment for a recall examination and cleaning. The receptionist, Ms. Nakanishi, answers the phone.

Ms. Nakanishi（N） Valley Dental Clinic. ① May I help you?

Ms. Hernandez（H） I would like to make an appointment.

N Is this for a regular examination or do you have a problem that needs immediate attention?

H My name is Laura Hernandez ② and I just received a recall card from Dr. Takeuchi for my regular examination and cleaning.

N Hello Ms. Hernandez. ② The doctor will be delighted to see you. When would you like to come in?

H Is next Friday morning ③ OK?

N Yes. The doctor could see you at 9:30, ④ and Ms. Kimura could do your cleaning at 9:45. ⑤

H Is it possible to come a bit later? ⑥ I have to drop the children off at school. ⑦

① Central Dental Clinic	Pacific Dental Clinic
② Lisa Jackson	(Your name)
③ tomorrow evening	Thursday afternoon
④ 7:15pm	3:45pm
⑤ 7:30pm	4:00pm
⑥ earlier	earlier
⑦ fix dinner for my children	see my friend at 4:00pm

（Pair Work 参照）

263-00488

N Would 10:45 ⑧ be acceptable?

H That would be fine.

N We are looking forward to seeing you, then,
Friday, November 30, at 10:45. ⑨

H Thank you very much.

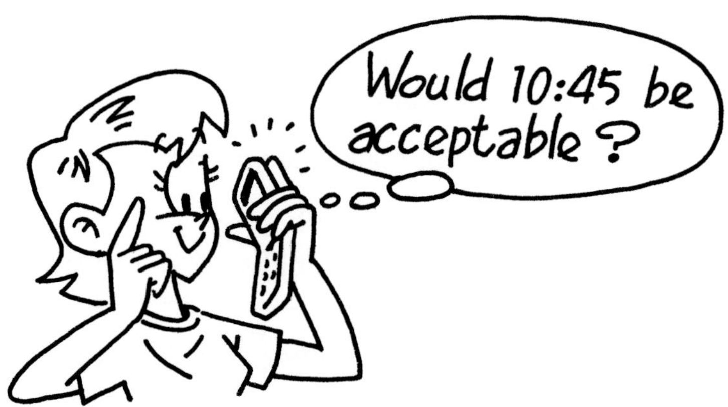

⑧	5:30pm	2:00pm
⑨	tomorrow, February 20, at 5:30pm	Thursday, August 5, at 2:00pm

（Pair Work 参照）

263-00488

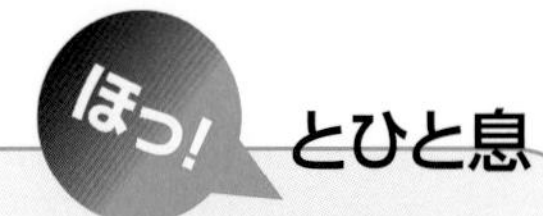

海外で活躍する歯科衛生士　1

岡山歯科衛生専門学校（現 朝日医療大学校歯科衛生学科）卒
山本祐子

●海外への夢

私が歯科衛生士学校に入学したころは，「世界をまたにかけて活躍する」という言葉をよく耳にする時代で，私も「歯科衛生士として海外で活躍したい」と思うようになりました．まだネットが普及していなかったので，過去の『デンタルハイジーン』を全部借りて関連記事の著者に手紙を書いたり，記事に出てきた施設について調べるなどして情報収集を行いました．

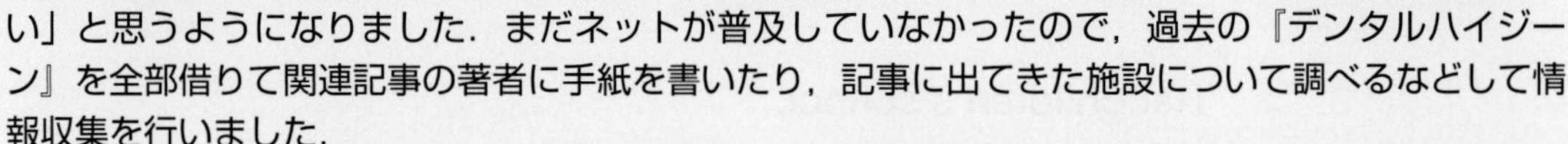

歯科衛生士学校卒業後，医療従事者を対象にした欧州福祉制度見学の研修に参加する機会を得ました．ここで「海外でも歯科衛生士として十分やっていける」手ごたえを感じ，本格的に渡航準備を始めました．行き先は英語圏で，以前より「歯科医療で先端を行っている」という感触を得ていた米国に焦点を絞ることにしました．

●歯科衛生士が評価される国･･･

その後，J1ビザ（研修生ビザ）を取得し，ニューヨークの歯科医院で助手として働くことができました．米国では，歯科衛生士が個室をもって患者さんの予約から処置のすべてを行い，初診の診察という責任の大きい役割も担っていました．「患者さんも歯科医師も歯科衛生士を高く評価している」，そんな光景に触れ，さらに米国への憧れが膨らみました．そんなとき出会ったのがいまの夫でした．

2年間帰国した後，再びニューヨークへ行って結婚，本格的にニューヨークでの生活が始まりました．しかし，ここで言葉の壁に直面しました．J1研修中に日常会話レベルの英語は身につけていたにもかかわらず….米国で英語ができないのは人格がないのと同じこと，そこで英語力をつけようと語学学校へ通ったところ，転機が訪れました．

●米国の大学に入学

語学学校で論文の書き方などを教わりおもしろさを感じ始めたときに，先生から大学入学をすすめられたのです．はじめは「普通の主婦に」と思っていたのに，夫の後押しもあって最終的にニューヨーク大学に入学することになってしまいました．

大学の講義は，習ったことのない内容ばかりで，興味深くおもしろいものでした．医療専門用語がラテン語で，覚えるのが大変だったり，英語が早口のため講義を録音して勉強しなおしたりと苦労もしましたが，とても刺激的でした．学生どうしによる実践中心の授業にも驚きで，入学直後から器材を用いて演習をするので，「患者さんにこんな痛い思いをさせたくない」と感じることもできました．実技テストはとても緊張したのですが，合格して最初にみる患者さんが家族や恋人なので，勉強の成果をみてもらえるというよろこびもありました．

現在は学校を卒業し臨床を続けていますが，今後は興味のある「食」に関する勉強をして歯科の仕事に活かしていきたいと思っています．

●学生へのメッセージ

歯科衛生士を目指しながら，同時に英語を勉強するのは容易なことではありませんが，堅苦しく考えずに楽しく学んで下さい．外国の文化，現地の人や食に興味をもつと英語の習得がグンと加速します．外国人に慣れ，片言の英語でも話す度胸を身につけることも大切ですよ．

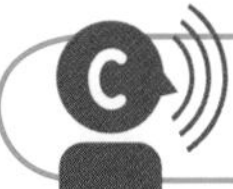

Listening 質問を聞いて，正しい答えを選びましょう

音声：01-L.mp3

1. *a* Because she needs immediate attention for her cavity.
   b Because she received a recall card for her regular examination.
   c Because she wants the doctor to see her children.

2. *a* Her children's school.
   b The doctor.
   c Another dental clinic.

3. *a* Because she has a problem with her children.
   b Because she needs to pick up her children at school.
   c Because she has to take her children to school.

4. *a* At 9:30 am
   b At 9:45 am
   c At 10:45 am

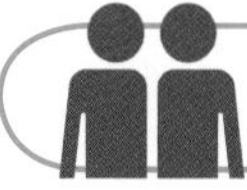

Pair Work

ペアになり，下線部を入れ替えて Dialogue を練習しましょう．

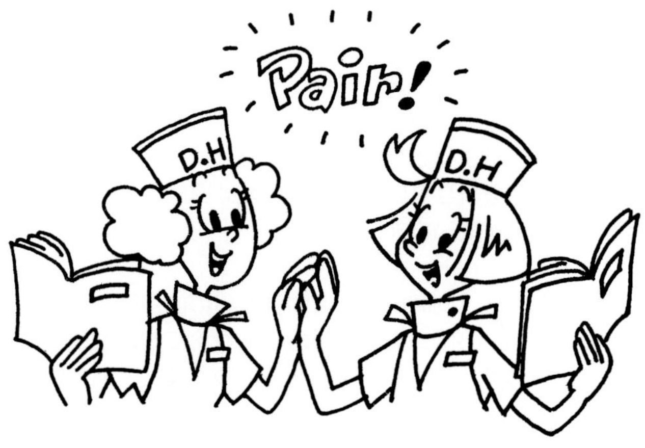

263-00488

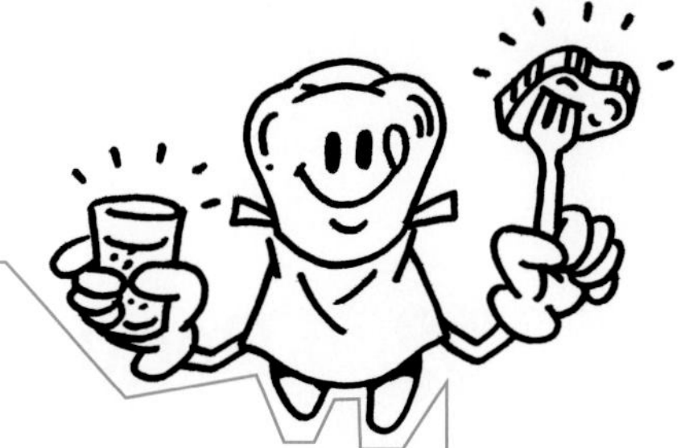

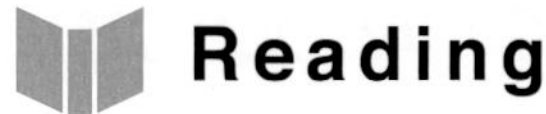

Reading

Healthy snacks for teeth（歯と栄養）

Snacks are an important part of many young children's diet. Children's energy needs are high, and they usually can't eat a lot at any one time like adults can. It is difficult for children to get all the nutrients they need to promote growth and development in three meals a day. Nearly all children eat at least one snack per day, with many children eating two or three. Snack foods provide the necessary calories for quickly growing young children. Healthy snacks will help supply all the nutrients like vitamins and minerals they require every day.

Snacking is good for pre-school and school-age children, but all snacks are not the same. Because snacks can provide a substantial amount of a child's food intake, they should be nutritious. The snacks we serve should be chosen carefully. It is a good idea to consider snacks as "mini meals" rather than treats, and make these foods a valuable part of the overall diet. Foods that promote good general health also promote good oral health. Try to establish both healthy eating patterns and daily dental care at an early age. Many dental professionals agree that for good dental health, some snack foods should be controlled and eaten sensibly. The source of the problem is sugar. Plaque, a sticky colorless layer of germs, will react with any sugar in your child's food to form acids which cause tooth decay.

How often and when certain foods are eaten influence the development of tooth decay. Eating between meals lengthens the amount of time the teeth are at risk. Avoid giving your child food and drinks between meals. Don't encourage a sweet tooth by adding sugar to snack foods and drinks, opt for low sugar brands of food, drinks and medicines. If your child does get hungry between meals, provide milk, fresh fruit, vegetables, cheese, yogurt, peanuts or eggs. Only give sweet foods and drinks at meal times and never a sweet drink before bedtime.

There are substances in our mouth which work for us to neutralize the acids and protect our teeth. However, every time food or drink enters our mouth the acidity caused by its reaction with plaque remains high for around half an hour and can take up to 2 hours to return to the normal level. If oral hygiene is poor, excessive snacking foods containing sugar may promote tooth decay. Restricting the number of between-meal snacks, including sweets, is an important way to reduce the potential risk of dental caries.

Q1　Are snacks fine for children?
Q2　What advice would you give to a mother about snacking?
Q3　Please describe healthy snacks.

263-00488

2 Requests for Medicine

Warm up

People will often ask for antibiotics or pain killers over the phone even though they have not visited the office. It is very irresponsible to give medicine to a patient without a proper examination and diagnosis. The patient must first be seen by the dentist.

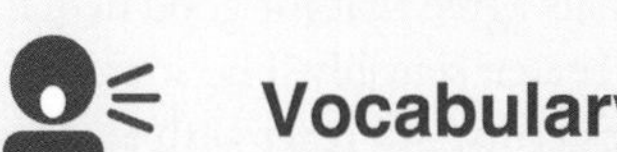

Vocabulary

antibiotic 〈名〉抗生物質
pain pill / pain killer 〈名〉鎮痛剤
irresponsible 〈形〉無責任な
tourist 〈名〉観光客
prescribe 〈動〉処方する *cf.* prescription 処方箋
toothache 〈名〉歯の痛み
certainly 〈副〉もちろん，確実に

263-00488

Dialogue

音声：02-D.mp3

Situation Mr. DiRisio is an Italian tourist who is on vacation in Japan. The receptionist, Ms. Goto, is explaining why the dentist cannot prescribe medicine without doing an examination.

Ms. Goto（G） Kanto Dental Clinic. ① May I help you?

Mr. DiRisio（D） I have a toothache, but I am too busy ② to come to your office. What should I do to stop it?

G The dentist must first examine ③ the tooth before he can decide the best treatment.

D But I am only in Japan for two weeks ④ and I have to go to Kyoto today. I am very busy.

G I understand your situation, but the dentist can't prescribe medicine without first doing an examination and diagnosis.

D I guess I will just have to come to your office.

G The dentist can see you at 10:30 ⑤ this morning and examine the tooth if you like.

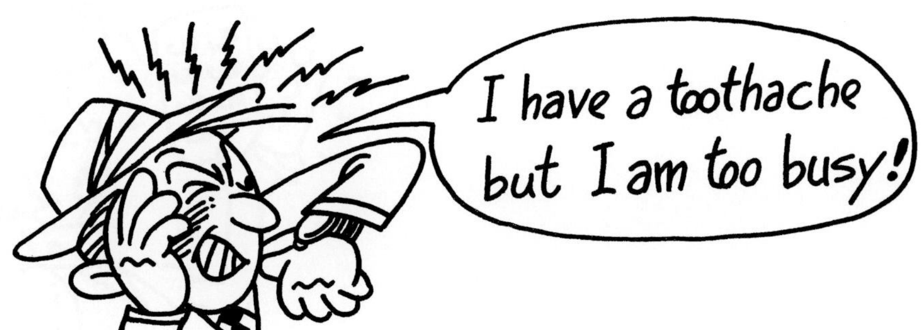
I have a toothache but I am too busy!

①	Yokohama Dental Clinic	Chiba Dental Clinic
②	don't have time	am not able
③	check	see
④	one week	ten days
⑤	9:30	11:30

（Pair Work 参照）

263-00488

D I will be there at 10:30. ⑥

G Could I have your name and phone number?

D Certainly. My name is Fabrizio DiRisio ⑦ and I am in Room 45325 ⑧ at the Grand Hyatt.

G Thank you Mr. DiRisio ⑨. We will see you at 10:30. ⑥

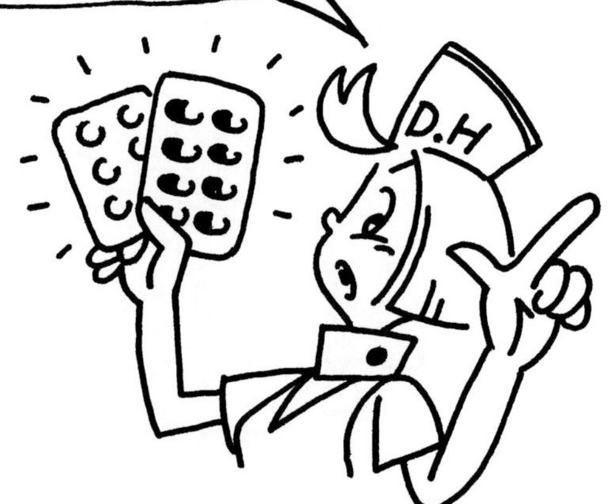
The dentist can't prescribe medicine without first doing an examination and diagnosis.
D.H

⑥	9:30	11:30
⑦	(Your name)	(Your name)
⑧	60523	17908
⑨	(Other party's name)	(Other party's name)

(Pair Work 参照)

263-00488

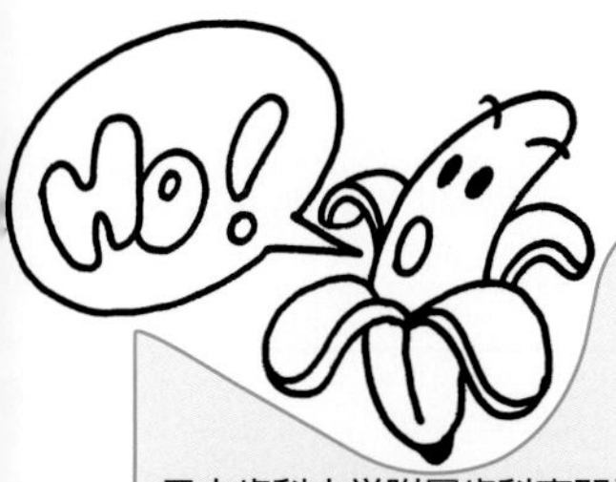

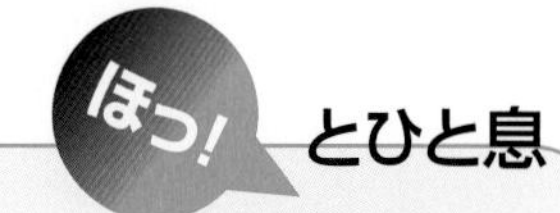

海外で活躍する歯科衛生士　2

日本歯科大学附属歯科専門学校歯科衛生士科（現 日本歯科大学東京短期大学歯科衛生学科）卒
星野由香里

●スウェーデンへの憧れ

スウェーデンへの憧れが芽生えたのは，日本歯科大学附属病院勤務中にスウェーデンのLindhe教授の講演を何度か受講し，スウェーデンの歯科衛生士の仕事に感銘を受けたと同時に，実際にどのように歯周病の患者さんが診られているのかを知りたいと思うようになったからです．その後，1週間のスウェーデン海外研修に参加する機会を得て，スウェーデンの歯科衛生士の仕事ぶりに触れてからはますますその想いが強くなりました．しかし，せっかくスウェーデンの歯科衛生士に対面できたものの，英語がわからず会話もままなりませんでした．「あー，言葉がわかればもっといろいろなことが聞けたのに」という悔しい思いをし，これをきっかけに「英語を習おう」と心に決めました．

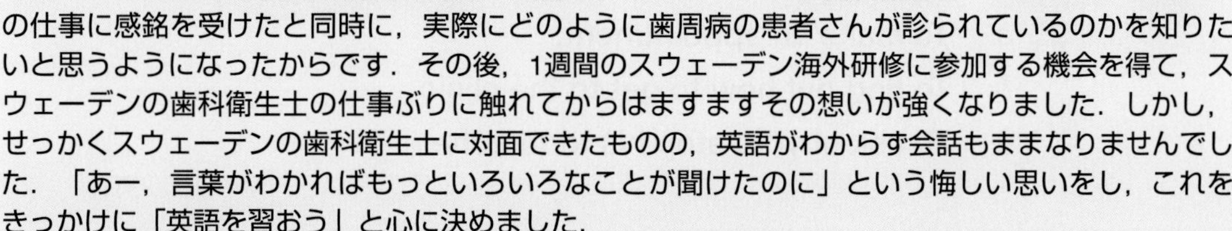

すぐに英会話教室に申し込んだものの，最初は仕事帰りで疲れているとついサボってしまい，決して熱心ではありませんでした．そんなとき，現奥羽大学教授の岡本　浩先生から「2年間スウェーデンで歯科衛生士の仕事を勉強してこないか」とすすめられました．「是非行きたい」と思っていたのですぐに承諾しました．スウェーデンの受け入れ先と勤務先の日本歯科大学の許可を得ましたが，留学まで約1年たらず．そこからは，週3回の個人レッスンにまじめに通ったり，電車のなかで英語のテープを聴いたりと，英語の猛勉強が始まりました．目標があることの効果に自分でも驚かされました．

●いざスウェーデンへ

スウェーデンに行ってみると，周りはみな外国人(本当は，私が外国人)ばかりで，あがってしまって話しかけられても口がパクパクしている状態でした．きちんとした文章でしゃべろうとすると余計言葉が出てこないのです．そんなとき，友人に「別に単語だけでも通じるよ，コミュニケーションをとることが大切なんだよ」と教えられました．「たとえば『どこからきたの』と聞かれたときに，『日本』と答えるだけで立派に会話になるでしょ」と．目からうろこが落ちる思いでした．

それからは，少しリラックスできるようになったものの，なかなか仲間に入れてもらえずさびしく感じることが多々ありました．しかし，自分から積極的に話しかけることで，みんなのなかに入っていくことができました．文化の違いもあり，ただ待っているだけでは誰も助けてくれないのです．わからないときは笑ってごまかさず，はっきりわからないということが大切なのです．

この2年間の留学で，歯科衛生士の仕事の大切さやおもしろさを教えられたのと同時に，人とのコミュニケーションの大切さ，さまざまな考え方や文化についても学ぶことができました．そのお陰か，帰国後は楽しんで仕事ができるようになりました．

●英語が可能性を広げます

1994年，再度スウェーデンで働くというチャンスに恵まれ，日本から離れることになりました．海外で歯科衛生士として働くためには，まずその国のライセンスを取得しなければならないのですが，そのためにはその国の言葉ができることが必須です．また，その国の人以上に頑張らないと認めてもらうのが難しいと感じています．

近年，主人の仕事の関係で米国・ボストン市（マサチューセッツ州）に1年半ほど滞在しました．このとき歯科研究機関で研修することができたのですが，これも歯科衛生士をやっていたおかげです．日本国内だけでなく海外の人とも出会うことのできる仕事ってよいと思いませんか？　そのためには，英語をやってて損はなし，チャンスがもっと広がると思いますよ．

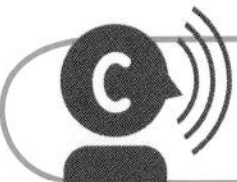

Listening 質問を聞いて，正しい答えを選びましょう

音声：02-L.mp3

1. *a* Studying.
   b Working.
   c Traveling.

2. *a* To make an appointment.
   b To find out how to get to the clinic.
   c To ask how to stop his toothache.

3. *a* Check the tooth.
   b Prescribe medicine.
   c Have his name and phone number.

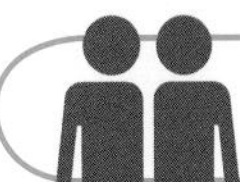

Pair Work

ペアになり，下線部を入れ替えて Dialogue を練習しましょう．

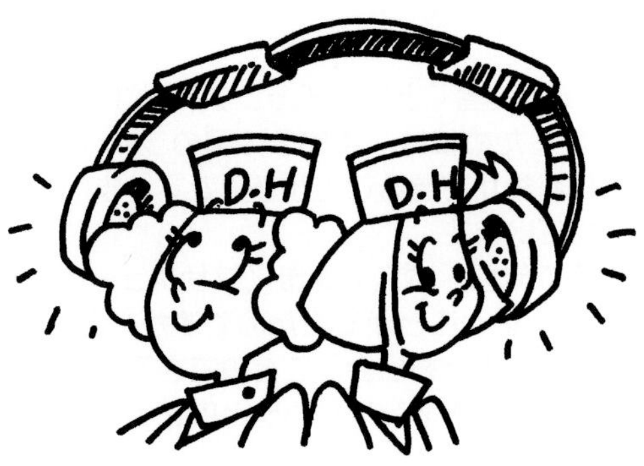

263-00488

Reading

Toothbrush and brushing（歯ブラシと歯磨き）

Why do you brush your teeth?

Brushing your teeth is one of the most effective ways of removing plaque and the large food particles that get trapped between your teeth. However, most people do not brush their teeth appropriately. They tend to spend too little time for brushing, and consistently miss certain parts of their teeth. As plaque accumulates, it becomes a major contributor to tooth decay and gum disease, the two most common dental diseases.

Plaque is an almost invisible sticky film formed from millions of bacteria. If not removed, the bacteria in plaque feed on food left in your mouth, and produce decay acids that eat into the enamel and thereby cause dental cavities. The plaque also acts on your gum tissues causing gum disease. Correct brushing helps prevent tooth cavities and gum disease. Change your toothbrush once the bristles get crushed or start to spread - with proper use, every 2 or 3 months.

What kind of toothbrush is best to use?

With so many shapes, sizes and styles of toothbrushes on the market, deciding which toothbrush to use can be confusing. You should have the right toothbrush as it will make brushing easier and more effective. It should have soft bristles with rounded ends and conform to individual variations in tooth-gum structures. A gentle brushing with a soft-bristle toothbrush is just as effective as a large scrubbing with a hard-bristle toothbrush.

The head should be small enough to reach all the surfaces of your teeth. The neck should be long and slim, so you can get to your back teeth and between the tongue and lower back teeth properly. A large brush doesn't efficiently get on to areas where dental plaque stagnates. The handle should be comfortable to hold, for better control when you brush.

The tooth enamel is relatively thin. Years of aggressive brushing with a hard bristle toothbrush can begin to wear away the enamel and make the teeth sensitive. The enamel on your teeth does not contain nerve fibers, but the dentin layer underneath does. Brushing too hard with a poor quality toothbrush can also damage your delicate gums.

Q1 What kind of toothbrush do you use?
Q2 Have you ever used an interdental brush?
Q3 What will happen if I brush my teeth with a hard bristle toothbrush and strong power?

263-00488

3 Emergency Appointments

Warm up

People will often ask for a diagnosis and cost estimate over the telephone. It is not possible to make a diagnosis or treatment plan until an examination has been done.

Vocabulary

toothache 〈名〉歯の痛み ***cf.*** headache 〈名〉頭痛
stomachache 〈名〉腹痛
describe 〈動〉描写する，説明する
symptom 〈名〉症状，徴候
molar 〈名〉大臼歯，奥歯
throb 〈動〉ズキズキ痛む
tooth 〈名〉歯 ***cf.*** 複数形は teeth
extract 〈動〉抜く（= pull）
relieve 〈動〉和らげる，楽にさせる
cost 〈動〉費用がかかる ***cf.*** 〈名〉費用
inform ～ of … 〈動〉～に…を知らせる
procedure 〈名〉手順，処置

Dialogue

音声：03-D.mp3

Situation Mr. Moore is requesting an emergency appointment for a toothache. The receptionist, Ms. Tanaka, is answering the call.

Ms. Tanaka（T） Sennan International Dental Clinic. ① May I help you?

Mr. Moore（M） I have a bad toothache. Could I talk with the dentist?

T I am very sorry. He is with a patient and cannot come to the phone.

M But I need to see him as soon as possible.

T The dentist can see you this morning. But first could you describe your symptoms? ②

M The back molar on the upper right ③ side began throbbing as the plane was landing at Kansai International Airport yesterday.

T Are you taking any medications?

M I took pain pills, but they didn't help. What is the dentist going to do?

T He will first have to do an examination and take an X-ray.

M Will he pull ④ the tooth?

T Dr. Suzuki does not like to extract teeth. He prefers to save them. But first he will do treatment to relieve the pain.

---

① Osaka Central Dental Clinic	Kobe International Dental Office
② discomfort	problem
③ the lower right	the upper left
④ remove	get rid of

（Pair Work 参照）

M That is what I want. How much will it cost?

T The cost of the treatment depends on what is done. He will first have to examine the tooth. The doctor never does treatment without informing you of ⑤ the procedure and cost.

M How much does the examination cost?

T The examination and X-ray will be 10,000 yen. ⑥

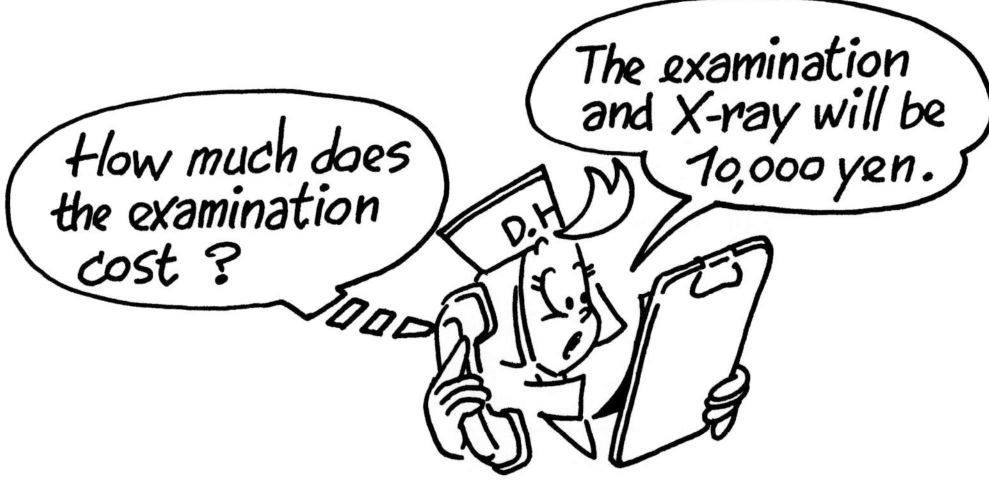

⑤ telling you　　letting you know

⑥ 13,500 yen　　11,700 yen

(Pair Work 参照)

263-00488

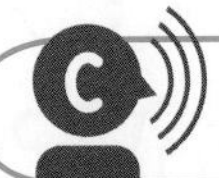

Listening 質問を聞いて，正しい答えを選びましょう

音声：03-L.mp3

1. *a* Because he doesn't like to talk with patients.
   b Because he is out for lunch at the moment.
   c Because he is busy with another patient.

2. *a* While he was waiting for a plane at Kansai Airport.
   b While he was on a plane approaching Kansai Airport.
   c While he was driving to Kansai Airport.

3. *a* Where the clinic is located and how long it would take from Kansai Airport.
   b What kind of treatment he will receive and how much he will have to pay.
   c How he could reduce the toothache without taking pain pills.

4. *a* Examine Mr. Moore's tooth using an X-ray.
   b Extract Mr. Moore's tooth and decide what to do next.
   c Give Mr. Moore some advice as to what pain pills to take.

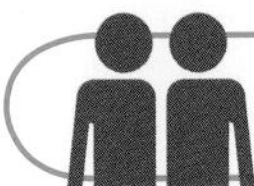

Pair Work

ペアになり，下線部を入れ替えて Dialogue を練習しましょう.

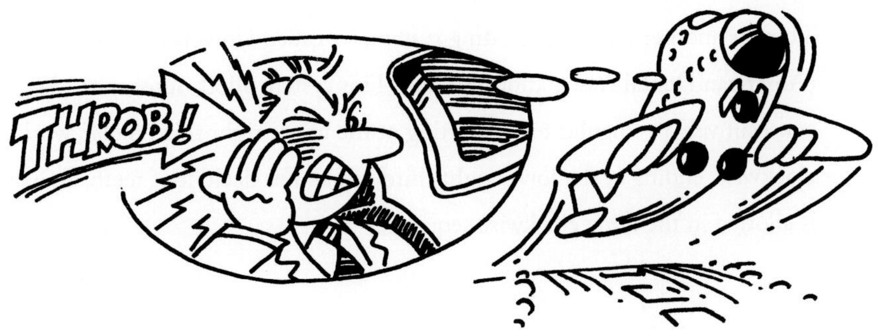

263-00488

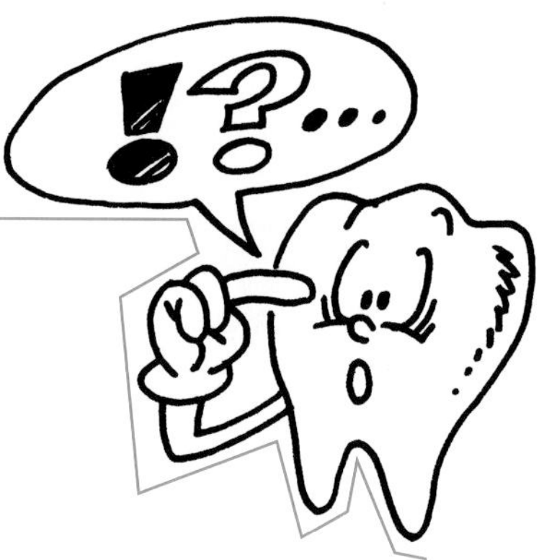

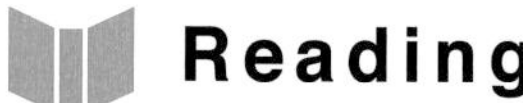

Reading

Tooth designating system（歯式）

In Japan, we use angular or grid system for designating teeth. For example, an upper right first molar is written in the form of 6|. This system is called the Palmer system.

However in the world, most countries adopt the Two-Digit System for designating teeth. According to the Two-Digit System, the first digit indicates the quadrant and the second digit indicates the type of tooth within the quadrant. Quadrants are allotted the digits 1 - 4 for the permanent teeth and 5 - 8 for the deciduous teeth in a clockwise sequence and starting at the upper right side. Teeth within the same quadrant are allotted the digits 1 - 8 for permanent teeth and 1 - 5 for the deciduous teeth from midline backwards. The digits should be pronounced separately. For example, first molars are teeth one-six, two-six, three-six and four-six.

The advantages of using Two-Digit System are the followings:
(1) Simple to understand and to teach
(2) Easy to pronounce in conversation and dictation
(3) Readily communicable in print and by wire
(4) Easy to translate into computer "input"
(5) Easily adaptable to standard charts used in general practice

There is another tooth designating system, so-called Universal System or ADA (American Dental Association) System. This system allots numbers 1 - 32 consecutively to singular teeth, starting at the upper right third molar, working clockwise, ending at the lower right third molar. For deciduous teeth, alphabet A-T is allotted in the same clockwise sequence.

263-00488

Palmer system

Permanent teeth

upper right	upper left
8 7 6 5 4 3 2 1	1 2 3 4 5 6 7 8
8 7 6 5 4 3 2 1	1 2 3 4 5 6 7 8
lower right	lower left

Deciduous teeth

upper right	upper left
E D C B A	A B C D E
E D C B A	A B C D E
lower right	lower left

Two-Digit system

Permanent teeth

upper right	upper left
18 17 16 15 14 13 12 11	21 22 23 24 25 26 27 28
48 47 46 45 44 43 42 41	31 32 33 34 35 36 37 38
lower right	lower left

Deciduous teeth

upper right	upper left
55 54 53 52 51	61 62 63 64 65
85 84 83 82 81	71 72 73 74 75
lower right	lower left

ADA System

Permanent teeth

upper right	upper left
1 2 3 4 5 6 7 8	9 10 11 12 13 14 15 16
32 31 30 29 28 27 26 25	24 23 22 21 20 19 18 17
lower right	lower left

Deciduous teeth

upper right	upper left
A B C D E	F G H I J
T S R Q P	O N M L K
lower right	lower left

Q1 How do you describe a lower left second molar in two-digit system?

Q2 How do you describe an upper right cuspid in two-digit system?

Q3 How do you describe a lower right deciduous first incisor in two-digit system?

4 National Health Insurance

Warm up

Many foreigners living in Japan have Japanese National Health Insurance. It may be necessary to explain to them what it covers and how they can use it.

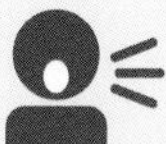

Vocabulary

National Health Insurance 〈名〉国民健康保険
treatment 〈名〉処置，治療
accept 〈動〉受け取る
crown 〈名〉クラウン
porcelain 〈名〉陶材
filling 〈名〉充填（物）*cf.* fill 〈動〉充填する，埋める
composite resin 〈名〉コンポジットレジン，合成樹脂

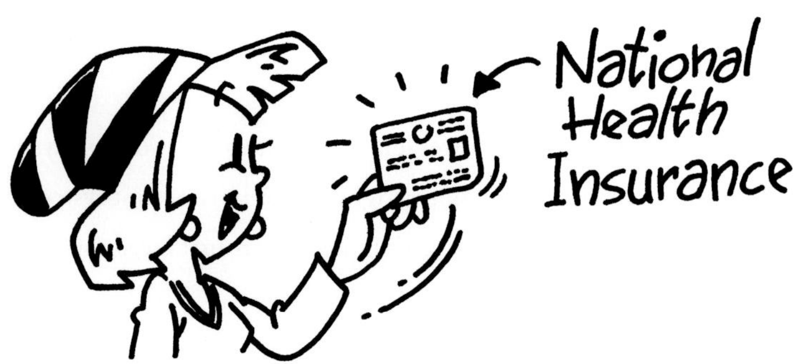

263-00488

Dialogue

音声：04-D.mp3

Situation Ms. Suharno, who is from Indonesia, recently received a Japanese National Health Insurance card and is asking the receptionist, Ms. Takeda, about treatment.

Ms. Suharno（S） I have a Japanese National Health Insurance card. Do you accept it?

Ms. Takeda（T） Yes, of course.

S Does it pay for all of my treatment?

T No. You have to pay about 30 % ① of the cost.

S Will the doctor tell me how much the treatment costs? ②

T Of course. He will always inform you before he does anything. If you have any questions, be sure to ③ ask him.

S Does the National Health Insurance pay for crowns? ④

T Yes, it covers crowns ④, but not porcelain crowns. ⑤

S How about white fillings?

T It covers composite resin fillings.

S What is that?

T Composite resin is half plastic and half glass. It looks just like the natural tooth.

S That's what I want. ⑥

① some	about one-third
② how long the treatment lasts	the treatment plan
③ don't hesitate to	feel free to
④ tooth extraction	dentures
⑤ orthodontic treatment	metal-plate denture
⑥ That sounds really good	I'd like to have that

（Pair Work 参照）

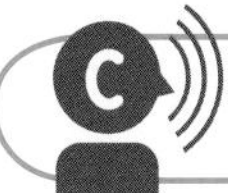

Listening 質問を聞いて，正しい答えを選びましょう

音声：04-L.mp3

1. *a* If she can use it for her treatment.
   b When her insurance card expires.
   c If she can get a new insurance card.

2. *a* His working hours.
   b His treatment policy.
   c His professional career.

3. *a* Porcelain crowns but not composite resin fillings.
   b Composite resin fillings but not porcelain crowns.
   c All types of crowns.

4. *a* A real tooth.
   b Plastic and glass.
   c A real tooth and plastic.

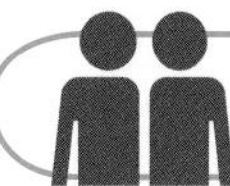

Pair Work

ペアになり，下線部を入れ替えて Dialogue を練習しましょう.

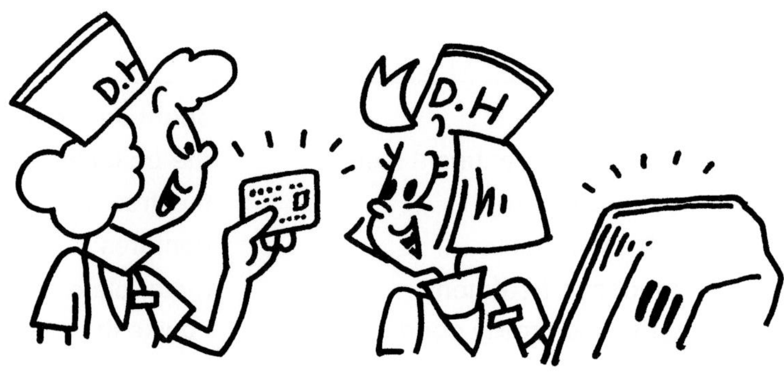

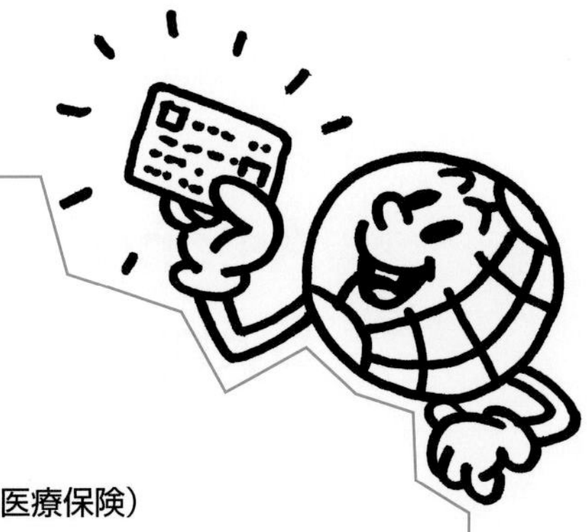

Reading

Insurance and expenditures for dental care（米国の歯科医療保険）

According to the U.S. Department of Health and Human Services, in 2002, the total expenditures for dental care in the U.S. were $70.3 billion or 4.5% of the total cost of personal health care expenditures. This represents an average per capita expenditure for dental care of $250. The expenditures for dental care as a percentage of the gross domestic product (GDP) were about 0.67%. Private sources, including private insurance and out-of-pocket spending by consumers, finance an overwhelming majority - 94% - of dental care expenditures. Payment by private insurance and direct consumer payment were 50% and 44%, respectively. Only over 6% of all dental expenditures were from public funds, primarily through the Medicaid programs where costs are shared jointly by the federal and state governments. The proportion of total public expenditures on health care services that went to dental care was less than 0.7%. The nearly $3.7 billion were paid by Medicaid for dental services. Besides the Medicaid program, other programs of public financing for dental care were provided by the Indian Health Service and the Health Resources and Services Administration. One of the major barriers to dental health includes socioeconomic factors, such as lack of dental insurance or the inability to pay out of pocket. Currently, many Americans do not have adequate insurance coverage. The number of children and adults without any type of dental insurance were more than 108 million - over 2.5 times the number without medical insurance (44 million). Only 60% of adults receive dental insurance through their employers, while most older workers lose their dental insurance at retirement. Meanwhile, uninsured children are 2.5 times less likely to receive dental care than insured children, and children from families without dental insurance are 3 times as likely to have dental needs compared to their insured counterparts.

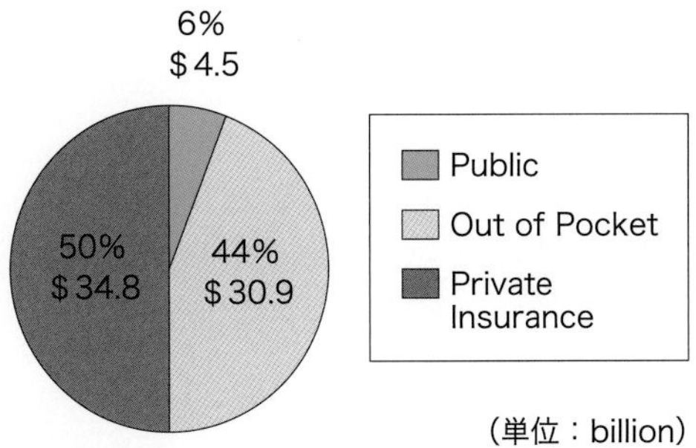

Proportion of total dental expenditures, by payers, 2002 (U.S. Department of Health and Human Services, Centers for Medicare and Medicaid Services, Highlights-National health expentidure, 2002. より)

Q1 Is the share of private dental finance bigger than that of public one?
Q2 How many Americans don't have dental insurance?
Q3 Please describe one of the major barriers to oral health.

5 Asking the Patient to Describe Symptoms

Warm up

Patients with dental emergencies may come when the doctor has a busy schedule. In order to help the doctor save time, the dental hygienist can ask the patient to describe his symptoms and report this to the doctor before he even sees the patient.

Vocabulary

symptom 〈名〉症状，徴候
dental hygienist 〈名〉歯科衛生士
bother 〈動〉悩ます，困らせる
irritate 〈動〉イライラさせる
sensitive 〈形〉敏感な
cavity 〈名〉むし歯
diagnosis 〈名〉診察，診断
discomfort 〈名〉不快，苦痛
painful 〈形〉痛い
chew 〈動〉かむ
appreciate 〈動〉感謝する，（価値などを）認識する

263-00488

Dialogue

音声：05-D.mp3

Situation Ms. Marsden has come to the clinic for treatment of a toothache. The dental hygienist, Ms. Sato, asks her a few questions about her condition to report to the dentist.

Ms. Sato（S） I understand that you have a toothache.

Ms. Marsden（M） Yes. My tooth is killing me.

S I would like to ask you a few questions so that I can report your situation to Dr. Murata.

M OK.

S First, which tooth is bothering you?

M It is on the lower right side, in back.

S Do you know exactly which tooth?

M I am not sure.

S How long has it hurt?

M It has been irritating me for several weeks, but it really got bad yesterday.

S Is it sensitive to hot or cold?

M First it was sensitive to cold, but now when I drink something hot it really throbs.

S Have you had any dental treatment recently?

M I had a crown put on the second tooth from the back a few months ago and the dentist said the cavity was very deep.

S That tooth might be the problem.

M What is the dentist going to do?

263-00488

S First he will take an X-ray and do a diagnosis. Then he will explain what needs to be done.

M OK.

S How about sweets? Do they cause discomfort?

M No. Not so much.

S Is the tooth painful when you chew?

M Yes. I have been chewing only on the left side for several days.

S I will report all of this to Dr. Murata and he will see you in a few minutes.

M Thank you. I really appreciate your help.

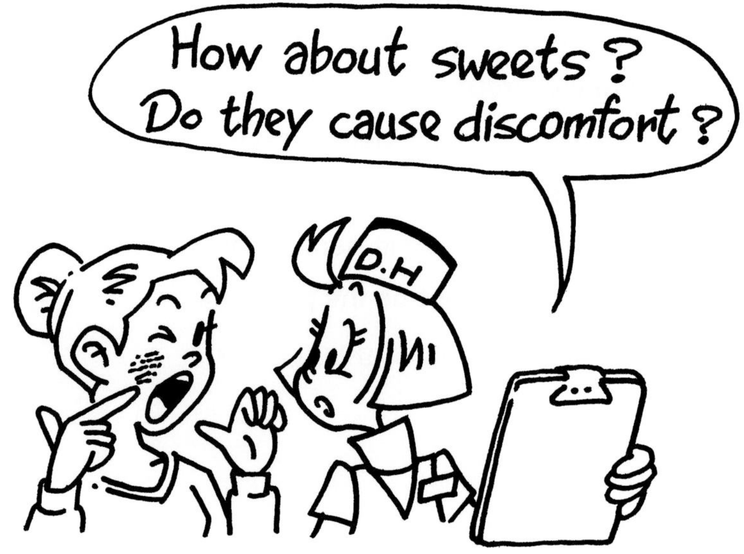

263-00488

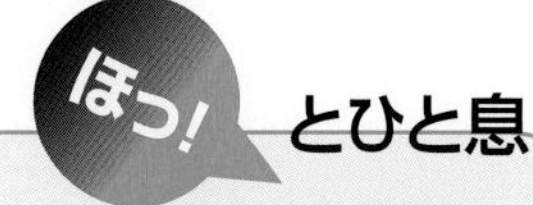

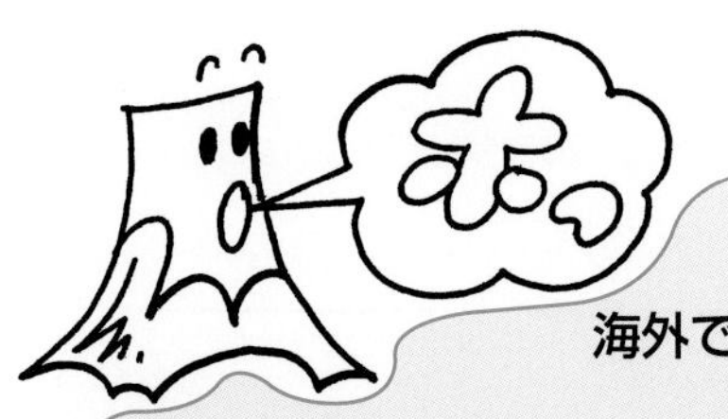

海外で活躍する歯科衛生士　3

愛知学院大学歯科衛生専門学校（現 愛知学院大学短期大学部歯科衛生学科）卒
足立弘美

●留学への夢

「海外旅行のときに英語で会話できたらいいな」　歯科衛生士として働き始めて数カ月後にそんな思いで通い始めた英会話学校でしたが，続けるほどに留学の望みが大きくなり，3年後には米国・コロラド州にわたっていました．当初は，言いたいことが英語で話せず，そのうえ発音が悪いために理解されず，もどかしく悔し涙の日々が続きました．また，私の通った大学は，日本人留学生が私一人だったので日本語が話せる人も少なく，ホームシックとの戦いでもありました．しかし，徐々に生活に慣れ，クラスメートや友人もでき，大学の先生方とも家族ぐるみで仲よくしてもらえたことで，よい思い出ができました．もちろん，勉強や国家試験では苦労しましたが……．おかげで念願がかない米国の歯科衛生士の資格をとることができました．

●米国の歯科衛生士について

米国の歯科衛生士の主な仕事内容は，エックス線写真撮影，OHI，浸潤麻酔，スケーリング・ルートプレーニングなどで，ドクターのアシスタントをすることは一切ありません．ドクターは私たち歯科衛生士の知識・技術を信頼しており，私たちの意見が治療方針にあたり重視されます．また，40代・50代の現役の歯科衛生士も多く，プロフェッショナルとして誇りをもって一生続けていくことができる職業です．

●英語学習のアドバイス

こちらに来て15年以上経ちますが，いまでもまだ知らない単語の意味を主人や友人に教えてもらったり，発音を直されたりします．英語を学ぶのは，簡単ではないけれど，はずかしがらず，失敗をおそれず，とにかく読んで，聞いて，話し続けると上達すると思います．また，正しく発音すること（特に日本人は，RとThの発音が苦手）を心がけることが大切です．さらに，英語から日本語に翻訳すると，意味やニュアンスが変わってしまう言葉などが理解できるようになると，もっと楽しくなると思います．

米国に来たことで，日本のよい点，悪い点を外からみることができ，自分の人生をプラスにしていくことができ，本当の自分をみつけられたような気がします．皆さんもこれから，いろいろチャレンジすることがあると思いますが，くじけず頑張ってください．

Good Luck to Future Dental Hygienists!

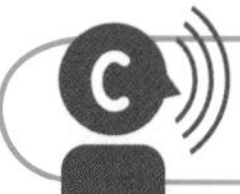

Listening 質問を聞いて，正しい答えを選びましょう

音声：05-L.mp3

1. *a* To help relieve the patient's pain.
   b To find out what problems the patient has.
   c To clean the patient's teeth.

2. *a* It became worse than before.
   b It became slightly better than before.
   c It didn't change at all.

3. *a* When she drinks something hot and chews something.
   b When she eats sweets and drinks something hot.
   c When she drinks something cold and sweet.

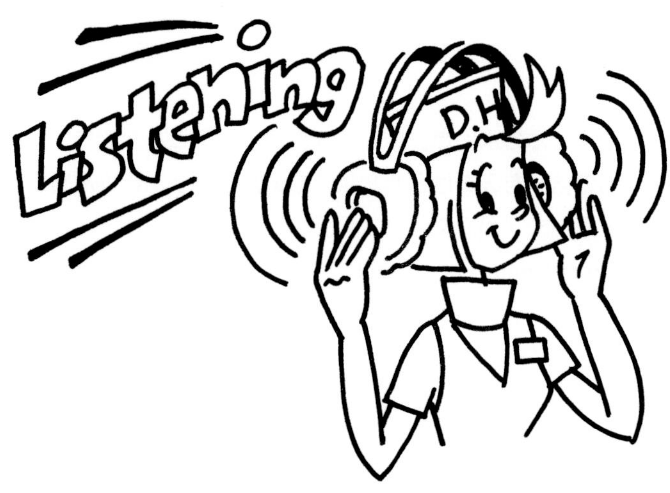

263-00488

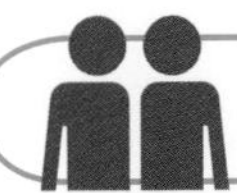

Pair Work

① まず自分が患者さんになったつもりで，以下の歯科衛生士の質問に対する自分なりの答えを考え，下線部に英語で書いてみましょう．次にペアになり，一人が歯科衛生士，もう一人が患者さんになってDialogue を練習しましょう．終わったら交代しましょう．

Dental Hygienist（DH） Which tooth is bothering you?

Patient（P）______________________________

DH Do you know exactly which tooth?

P ______________________________

DH How long has it hurt?

P ______________________________

DH Is it sensitive to hot or cold?

P ______________________________

DH Have you had any dental treatment recently?

P ______________________________

DH How about sweets? Do they cause discomfort?

P ______________________________

DH Is the tooth painful to chewing?

P ______________________________

② Dialogue のなかに出てきたもの以外で，患者さんの症状について歯科衛生士が聞いておくべき質問を一つ英語で書き，パートナーにたずねてみましょう．

質問 ______________________________?

パートナーの答え ______________________________

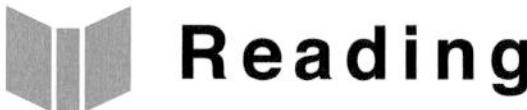

Reading

First aid steps for a knocked-out tooth（外傷による脱落歯の応急処置）

A tooth may be knocked out of the mouth as a result of an accident. With proper emergency action, the tooth that has been entirely knocked out of its socket can be successfully replanted and last for years. The best results occur if a dentist puts the tooth back in the socket within 30 minutes. Chances of successful replantation are unlikely after 2 hours. Because of this, it is important to be prepared and know what to do if this happens to you or someone around you. The following actions if carried out as promptly as possible may save the tooth.

1. Find the tooth.
Do not leave the tooth at the site of the accident. Apply clean gauze to the gum and socket to control the bleeding.

2. Handle the tooth by the crown not by the root.
The tooth should be handled carefully and touch only the crown (top of the tooth) to minimize injury to the delicate root. Handling the root may damage the cells necessary for bone re-attachment and hinder replacing the tooth.

3. If dirty, gently rinse the tooth with milk or water.
If the root has dirt on it, gently rinse the tooth with milk or water, remembering not to handle the root surface.

・Do not use cleaning agents, such as soap or chemicals.
・Do not vigorously rub or scrub the tooth.
・Do not dry the tooth.
・Do not wrap it in a tissue or cloth.

4. Immediately reposition the tooth in its socket, if possible.
The sooner the tooth is replaced, the greater the likelihood it will survive. To put the tooth back into the socket, gently place it back into its normal position with fingers, or position above the socket and bite down gently on gauze. Hold the tooth

263-00488

in place with fingers or by gently biting down on it during transport.

5. Store the tooth properly for transportation to the dentist.

The tooth must not be left outside the mouth to dry. However, it is possible to save the tooth even if it has been outside the mouth for an hour or more. If it cannot be replaced in the socket, put it in one of the following:

・Plastic wrap
・Milk
・Mouth (between the gums and the cheek or under the tongue)

If none of these is practical, use water. Do not put the tooth in salt water, alcohol, or mouthwash.

6. Seek dental help immediately within 30 minutes.

Bring the tooth to a dentist as soon as possible, ideally, within 30 minutes. It is essential that the tooth be replaced as quickly as possible.

Q1 Is it all right to pick up the root of the knocked-out tooth?
Q2 Is it better to clean the knocked-out tooth with toothpaste?
Q3 What is the method of protection of tooth injury during the sports?

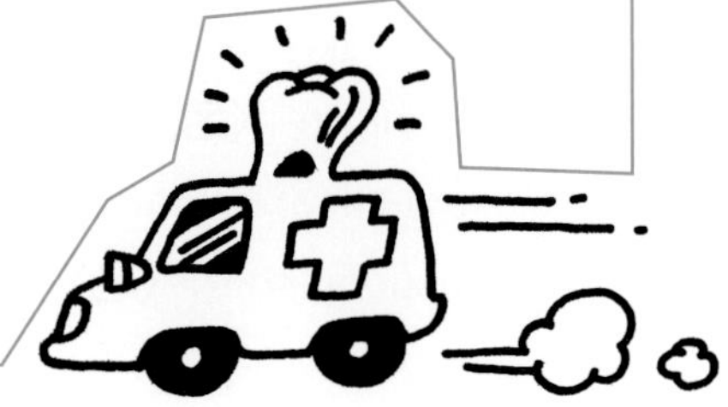

6 Asking the Medical History

Warm up

The dentist may request the dental hygienist to ask the patient about his medical history. What the patient says should be written down and given to the dentist. Any medical issues that the dental hygienist does not understand should be referred to the dentist.

Vocabulary

medical history 〈名〉病歴
examination 〈名〉検査
record 〈動〉記録する
affect 〈動〉影響を与える
gums 〈名〉歯肉
allergy 〈名〉アレルギー *cf.* allergic 〈形〉アレルギーの ※発音に注意
prescribe 〈動〉処方する *cf.* prescription 処方箋
cancer 〈名〉癌
recurrence 〈名〉再発
Tylenol 〈名〉タイレノール（米国で一般的な鎮痛剤）
anesthetic 〈名〉麻酔薬
penicillin 〈名〉ペニシリン
antibiotic 〈名〉抗生物質
root canal treatment 〈名〉根管治療
wisdom tooth 〈名〉親知らず（智歯）

263-00488

Dialogue

音声：06-D.mp3

Situation Mr. Mehta is coming to the clinic for his first visit. The dental hygienist, Ms. Abe, is reviewing his medical history before the examination by the dentist.

Ms. Abe（A） Dr. Shimizu has asked me to record your medical history.

Mr. Mehta（M） Why does he need that? I just want my teeth examined.

A Your medical condition can affect your teeth and gums.

M Really?

A Yes. Also, it is important for the doctor to know if you have any allergies or medical problems before he prescribes medicines.

M I understand.

A Have you ever had any serious illnesses?

M I had treatment for skin cancer twenty years ago, but there has been no recurrence.

A I see. Are you taking any medicines?

M Sometimes I take Tylenol when I have a headache.

A Do you have any allergies to medicines or dental anesthetics?

M Yes. I am allergic to penicillin. What will the doctor give me if I need an antibiotic?

A I am not sure. You should discuss that with him. I will make a note about this in your chart and he will ask you about it.

M Thank you.

A Have you had any extensive dental treatment, such as crowns or root canal treatment?

263-00488

M No. Only fillings.

A Have your wisdom teeth been extracted?

M Yes. All four of them were taken out ten years ago.

A I see. I will report this to Dr. Shimizu.

M Thank you.

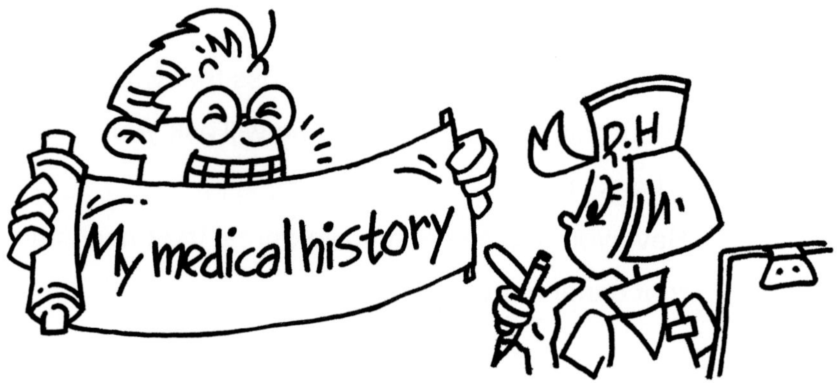

263-00488

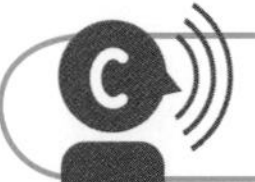

Listening 質問を聞いて，正しい答えを選びましょう

音声：06-L.mp3

1. *a* Because Ms. Abe wants to know what type of person Mr. Mehta is.
   b Because the cost of the treatment will be decided based on the patient's medical history.
   c Because the doctor must understand the patient's medical condition to avoid any problems during treatment.

2. *a* Medicines for skin cancer.
   b Pain killers occasionally.
   c No medicine.

3. *a* Tylenol.
   b Dental anesthetics.
   c Penicillin.

4. *a* Some pharmacist.
   b The dental hygienist.
   c The doctor.

5. *a* None.
   b One.
   c Two.

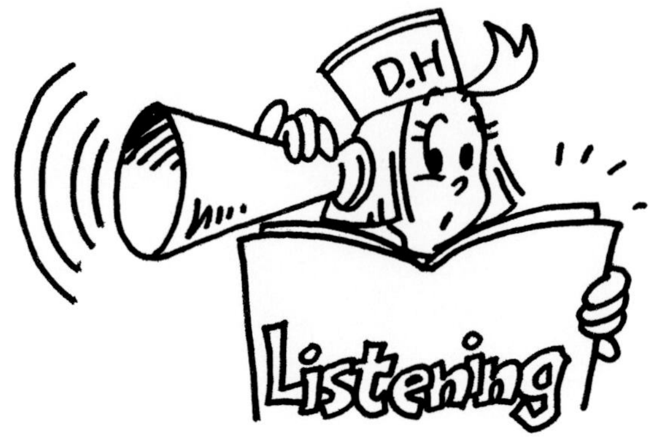

Pair Work

① まず自分が患者さんになったつもりで，以下の歯科衛生士の質問に対する自分なりの答えを考え，下線部に英語で書いてみましょう．次にペアになり，一人が歯科衛生士，もう一人が患者さんになってDialogue を練習しましょう．終わったら交代しましょう．

Dental Hygienist（DH） Have you ever had any serious illnesses?
Patient（P）＿＿＿＿＿＿＿＿＿＿＿＿＿＿＿＿＿＿＿＿
DH Are you taking any medicines?
P ＿＿＿＿＿＿＿＿＿＿＿＿＿＿＿＿＿＿＿＿
DH Do you have any allergies to medicines or dental anesthetics?
P ＿＿＿＿＿＿＿＿＿＿＿＿＿＿＿＿＿＿＿＿
DH Have you had any big dental treatments?
P ＿＿＿＿＿＿＿＿＿＿＿＿＿＿＿＿＿＿＿＿
DH Have your wisdom teeth been extracted?
P ＿＿＿＿＿＿＿＿＿＿＿＿＿＿＿＿＿＿＿＿

② Dialogue のなかに出てきたもの以外で，歯科衛生士として患者さんの病歴について聞いておくべき質問を一つ英語で書き，パートナーにたずねてみましょう．

質問 ＿＿＿＿＿＿＿＿＿＿＿＿＿＿＿＿＿＿＿＿?
パートナーの答え ＿＿＿＿＿＿＿＿＿＿＿＿＿＿＿＿＿＿＿＿

263-00488

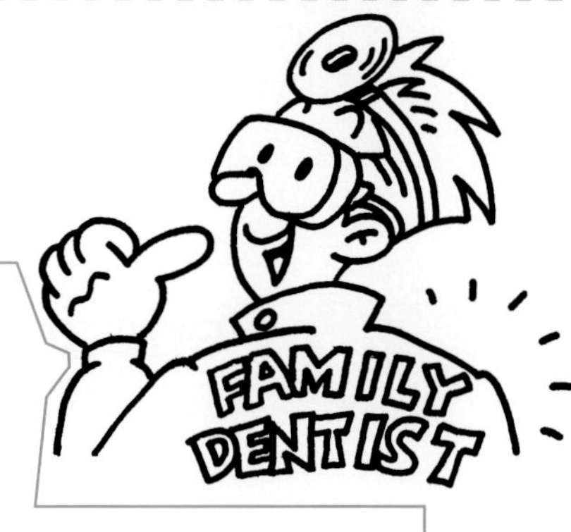

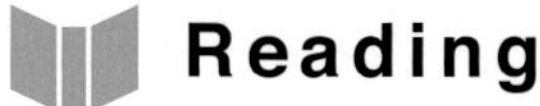

Health questionnaire（問診票）

Name ________________ Birthday (Day/Month/Year) ________ Sex : Male/ Female
Address ________________ Telephone number ________________

Please answer the following questions. They are helpful for your dental treatment.

Oral health

1. What is your oral problem? ________________
2. Are you receiving dental treatment now? Yes, No
3. When was your last visit to a dental clinic? ____year(s)/month(s) /day(s) ago
4. Have you ever had an injection for anesthesia? Yes, No
5. Have you ever had a tooth extraction? Yes, No
6. Have you ever had complications from dental treatment? Yes, No

General health

7. How is your health condition now? Excellent, Good, Poor
8. Are you under a doctor's care now? Yes, No
9. Do you have or have you ever had the following disease?
   Heart disease, Stomach disease, Kidney disease, Liver disease, Hepatitis, Hypertension, Hypotension, Anemia, Diabetes, Pneumonia, Asthma, Tuberculosis, Cancer, Blood disorder, Others(   )
10. Have you ever had an operation? Yes, No
11. Have you ever had a blood transfusion? Yes, No
12. Are you taking any medicines or drugs? Yes, No
13. Do you have an allergy? Yes, No
14. Do you smoke? Yes, No
15. Are you pregnant? Yes, No

Brushing behavior

16. How many times do you brush your teeth in a day? ______times
17. When do you brush your teeth? ________________
18. What kind of toothpaste do you use? ________________
19. Do you use dental floss or interdental brush? Yes, No
20. Do you brush your tongue? Yes, No

7 Periodontal Disease

Part I

Warm up

Dentists often ask the dental hygienist to explain periodontal disease to the patient. When explaining something like this, it helps the patient understand if you show a picture of what the tooth and gingiva look like.

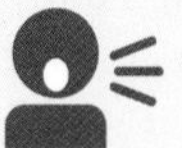

Vocabulary

periodontal disease 〈名〉歯周病
serious 〈形〉深刻な，真剣な
reverse 〈動〉逆転させる
drawing 〈名〉図面，図画
root 〈名〉歯根
bone 〈名〉骨
surround 〈動〉囲む
pocket 〈名〉歯周ポケット
calcium deposit 〈名〉カルシウム沈着物
tissue 〈名〉組織

263-00488

Dialogue

音声：07_Part1-D.mp3

Situation The dentist has asked the dental hygienist, Ms. Fujita, to explain periodontal disease to the patient, Mr. Garcia.

Ms. Fujita（F） Dr. Tanaka asked me to explain gum disease to you.

Mr. Garcia（G） It sounds serious. Is it really bad?

F Your case is in the early stages and can be reversed. However, if not treated, gum disease can cause the loss of teeth.

G I don't want to lose my teeth.

F I will make a drawing of a tooth to explain gum disease.

G Thank you. That would be helpful.

F This drawing is what the teeth and gums look like. The root of the tooth is as big as the part of the tooth above the gum line.

G I didn't know that.

F The gums and bone surround and support the tooth.

G I see.

F Between the gums and tooth is a pocket about one to three millimeters deep. When food, bacteria and calcium deposits get in this pocket, they can destroy the tissues that attach to the root.

G That sounds bad.

F It is bad. That's what causes gum disease.

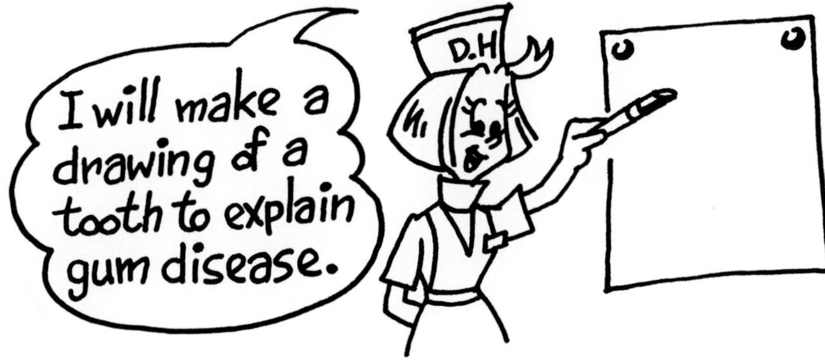

263-00488

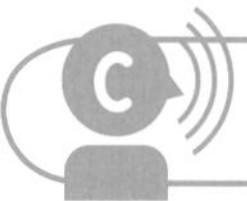

Listening 質問を聞いて，正しい答えを選びましょう

音声：07_Part1-L.mp3

1. *a* To clean Mr.Garcia's teeth.
   b To explain gum disease to Mr.Garcia.
   c To draw a picture of Mr.Garcia's gums.

2. *a* He would need to pay more.
   b He would lose his teeth.
   c He would get sick.

3. *a* Because she wanted to show Mr.Garcia that she is good at drawing.
   b Because Mr.Garcia requested her to do so.
   c Because she thought it would make her explanation clearer.

4. *a* Much smaller than the part of the tooth above the gum line.
   b About the same size as the part of the tooth above the gum line.
   c Much bigger than the part of the tooth above the gum line.

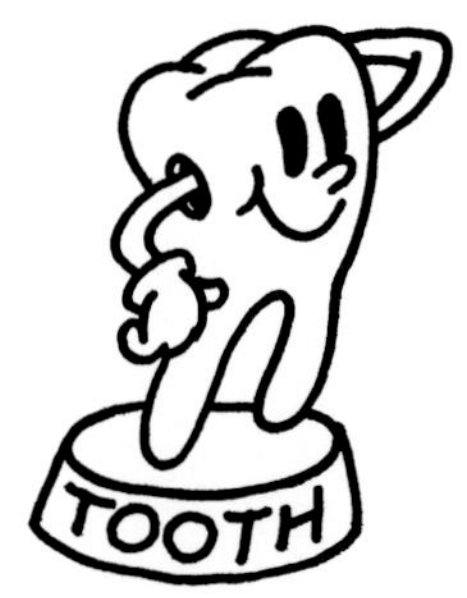

263-00488

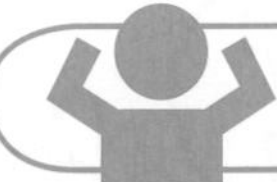

Exercise

Dialogue の内容を参考にして，実際に歯の絵を描いてみましょう.

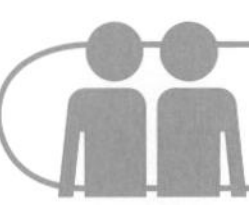

Pair Work

ペアになり，パートナーを患者さんと想定して歯周病について英語で説明してみましょう．終わったら交代しましょう.

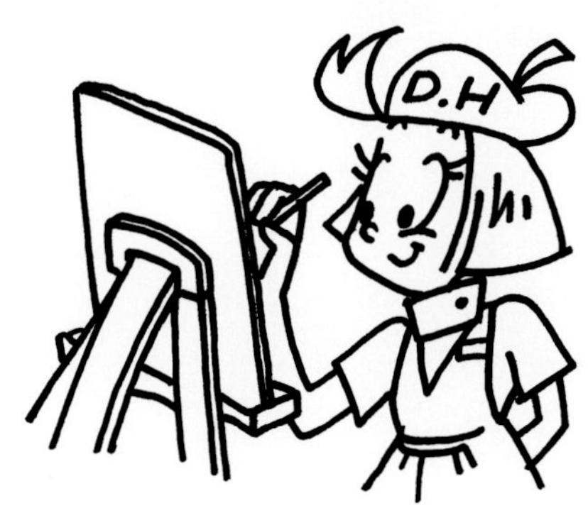

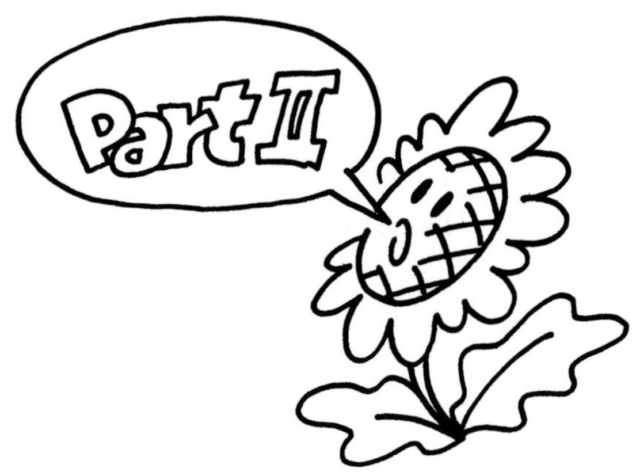

Part II

Warm up

This is a continuation of the previous dialogue.

Vocabulary

instrument 〈名〉器具
scaler 〈名〉スケーラー
remove 〈動〉取り除く
eliminate 〈動〉回避する，排除する
continue to ～ 〈動〉～し続ける
destroy 〈動〉壊す
loose 〈形〉ぐらついた，緩んだ

Dialogue

音声：07_Part2-D.mp3

Situation The dental hygienist explains to the patient how his periodontal condition will be treated.

Mr. Garcia（G） How will the doctor treat my gum disease?

Ms. Fujita（F） The first treatment is for me to use special instruments like this scaler.

G What is that?

F It is an instrument used to remove plaque and calcium deposits that are on the tooth, both above and below the gum line.

G How does that help?

F By doing this, the tissue around the teeth becomes healthy and gum disease can be eliminated.

G What if I don't do the treatment?

F Then the bacteria continue to destroy the tissues supporting the teeth.

G That sounds bad.

F It is. Bone will be destroyed and the teeth will become loose, like in this drawing.

G I don't want that.

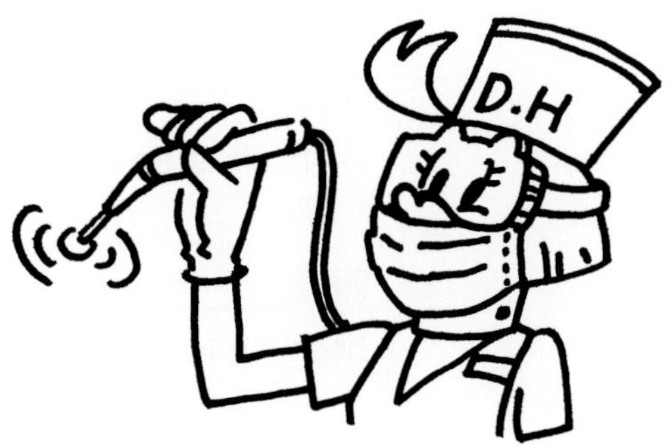

263-00488

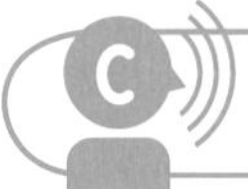

Listening 質問を聞いて，正しい答えを選びましょう

音声：07_Part2-L.mp3

1. *a* An instrument used to give brushing instructions.
   b An instrument used to get rid of plaque and calcium deposits.
   c An instrument used to draw a picture of a patient's teeth.

2. *a* Prevent gum disease.
   b Reduce the patient's pain.
   c Destroy the tissues around the teeth.

3. *a* The bacteria will be eliminated.
   b The bone will become weak.
   c The tissues will be healthy.

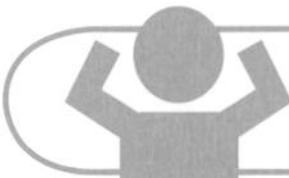

Exercise

例にならって歯科医療で使われる器具の用途について英語で説明しましょう.

（例） 器具 scaler
用途 It is an instrument used to remove plaque and calcium deposits that are on the tooth, both above and below the gum line.

① 器具 ______________________
用途 It is an instrument used to ______________________
____

② 器具 ______________________
用途 It is an instrument used to ______________________
____

③ 器具 ______________________
用途 It is an instrument used to ______________________
____

263-00488

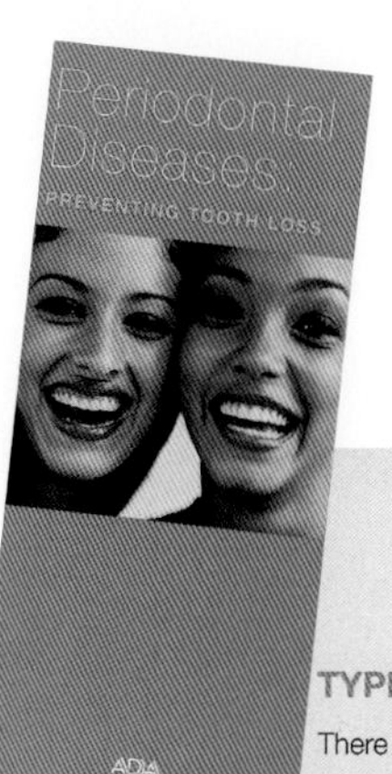

TYPES OF PERIODONTAL DISEASES

There are many types of periodontal diseases and they can affect individuals of all ages from children to seniors.

GINGIVITIS is the mildest form of periodontal disease. It causes the gums to become red, swollen, and bleed easily. There is usually little or no discomfort at this stage. Gingivitis is reversible with professional treatment and good oral care at home.

CHRONIC PERIODONTITIS is a form of periodontal disease that results in inflammation within the supporting tissues of the teeth. Patients experience progressive loss of tissue attachment and bone. Chronic periodontitis is characterized by pocket formation and/or recession of gum tissue and is the most frequently occurring form of periodontitis. It is prevalent in adults, but can occur at any age. Progression of attachment loss usually occurs slowly, but periods of rapid progression can occur.

AGGRESSIVE PERIODONTITIS is a highly destructive form of periodontal disease that occurs in patients who are otherwise clinically healthy. Common features include rapid loss of tissue attachment and destruction of bone. This disease may occur in localized or generalized patterns.

PERIODONTITIS AS A MANIFESTATION OF SYSTEMIC DISEASES
This form of periodontitis is associated with one of several systemic diseases, such as diabetes. Patients who have rare but specified blood diseases or genetic disorders frequently show signs of periodontal diseases.

NECROTIZING PERIODONTAL DISEASES are infections characterized by necrosis (death) of gingival tissues, periodontal ligament and alveolar bone. These lesions are most commonly associated with pain, bleeding, and a foul odor. Contributing factors can include emotional stress, tobacco use and HIV infection.

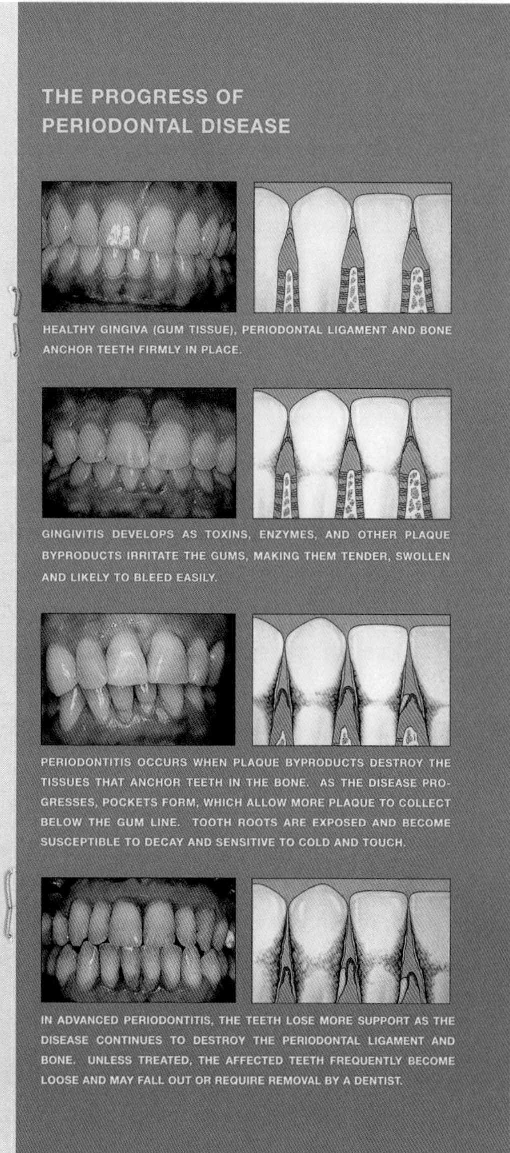

THE PROGRESS OF PERIODONTAL DISEASE

HEALTHY GINGIVA (GUM TISSUE), PERIODONTAL LIGAMENT AND BONE ANCHOR TEETH FIRMLY IN PLACE.

GINGIVITIS DEVELOPS AS TOXINS, ENZYMES, AND OTHER PLAQUE BYPRODUCTS IRRITATE THE GUMS, MAKING THEM TENDER, SWOLLEN AND LIKELY TO BLEED EASILY.

PERIODONTITIS OCCURS WHEN PLAQUE BYPRODUCTS DESTROY THE TISSUES THAT ANCHOR TEETH IN THE BONE. AS THE DISEASE PROGRESSES, POCKETS FORM, WHICH ALLOW MORE PLAQUE TO COLLECT BELOW THE GUM LINE. TOOTH ROOTS ARE EXPOSED AND BECOME SUSCEPTIBLE TO DECAY AND SENSITIVE TO COLD AND TOUCH.

IN ADVANCED PERIODONTITIS, THE TEETH LOSE MORE SUPPORT AS THE DISEASE CONTINUES TO DESTROY THE PERIODONTAL LIGAMENT AND BONE. UNLESS TREATED, THE AFFECTED TEETH FREQUENTLY BECOME LOOSE AND MAY FALL OUT OR REQUIRE REMOVAL BY A DENTIST.

（ADA: Periodontal Diseases. より）

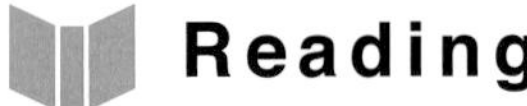

Reading

Tobacco and oral health（タバコと口腔保健）

It is estimated that there are 1.3 billion smokers in the world. Negative effects of tobacco on health such as lung cancer, heart disease and cerebral stroke are well-known. However those who consume tobacco are not the only ones exposed to its negative effects. Millions of people are exposed to second-hand tobacco smoke, known also as passive smoking.

Besides the damage on general health, tobacco consumption is related to oral diseases and other adverse conditions. For instance, smoking is a risk factor for oral cancer, periodontal diseases, gum melanosis and halitosis, and smoking decreases curative effect of dental treatments for periodontal diseases, dental implant and various surgical procedures. Furthermore, smokeless tobacco has been reported to be a risk factor of oral cancer, leukoplakia and other oral mucosa diseases.

Because smokers can directly see and recognize the symptom of tobacco-related oral diseases, it should be easy to motivate them to stop smoking and, thereby, prevent development of severe health hazards at early stage.

According to the national health and nutrition survey in 2003, current smoking rates in Japan are 46.8% in males and 11.3% in females. Since 1986, the smoking rate has tended to decrease but an increase of female and teenager smokers remain a big problem.

Dental professionals should be actively involved in tobacco control activities by providing appropriate oral health information in cooperation with other health professionals.

263-00488

The tobacco control efforts include the followings.

- To prevent people from taking up tobacco consumption
- To promote tobacco cessation
- To protect non-smokers from the exposure to tobacco smoke
- To regulate tobacco products

(Reference: The Role of Health Professionals in Tobacco Control (WHO))

Q1 What are negative effects of tobacco on general health?

Q2 What are negative effects of tobacco on oral health?

Q3 What are the smoking rate of Japanese males and females?

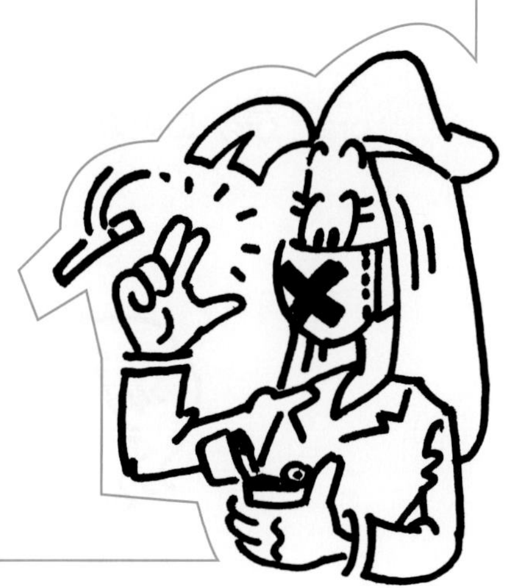

263-00488

8 Pregnancy

Warm up

The hormones associated with pregnancy can often make the gingiva swell and cause discomfort. Although this is not gum disease, it is important to maintain good oral health during pregnancy.

Vocabulary

pregnancy 〈名〉妊娠　*cf.* pregnant 〈形〉妊娠している
hormone 〈名〉ホルモン
associate … with ～ 〈動〉…を～と結びつける
swell 〈動〉腫れる　*cf.* swelling 〈形〉腫れている 〈名〉腫脹
discomfort 〈名〉不快，苦痛
maintain 〈動〉維持する，保つ
oral 〈形〉口腔の

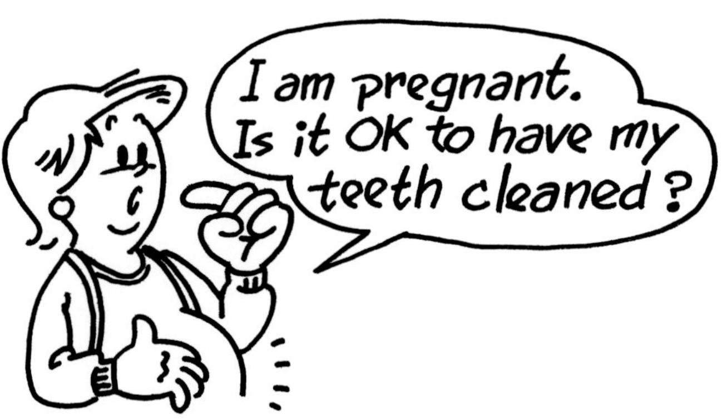
I am pregnant.
Is it OK to have my teeth cleaned?

263-00488

Dialogue

音声：08-D.mp3

Situation The dental hygienist, Ms. Otani, is explaining to a patient, Ms. Jansen, how pregnancy affects her oral health.

Ms. Jansen（J） I am pregnant. Is it OK to have my teeth cleaned?

Ms. Otani（O） There is no problem with having your teeth cleaned. In fact, it is important to maintain good dental health during pregnancy.

J Actually, my gums seem to be a bit uncomfortable recently.

O That often happens during pregnancy.

J Why is that?

O The hormones associated with pregnancy can cause the gums to swell.

J I didn't know that. Is it a problem?

O It is not serious, but you will feel more comfortable after your teeth are cleaned.

J Do I need to have X-rays?

O The doctor never takes X-rays when you are pregnant unless there is a serious condition.

J That's good. I would like to make an appointment as soon as possible.

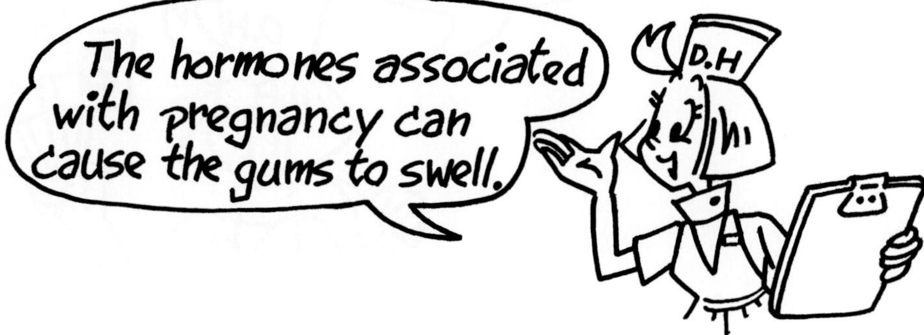

263-00488

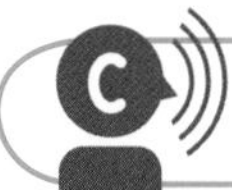

Listening 質問を聞いて，正しい答えを選びましょう

音声：08-L.mp3

1. *a* Whether it was OK to take pain killers during pregnancy.
   b Whether it was OK to have her teeth cleaned during pregnancy.
   c Whether it was OK to have her teeth extracted during pregnancy.

2. *a* Because of nutrition.
   b Because of diet.
   c Because of hormones.

3. *a* When she had a serious problem.
   b When she had a broken tooth.
   c When she had swollen gums.

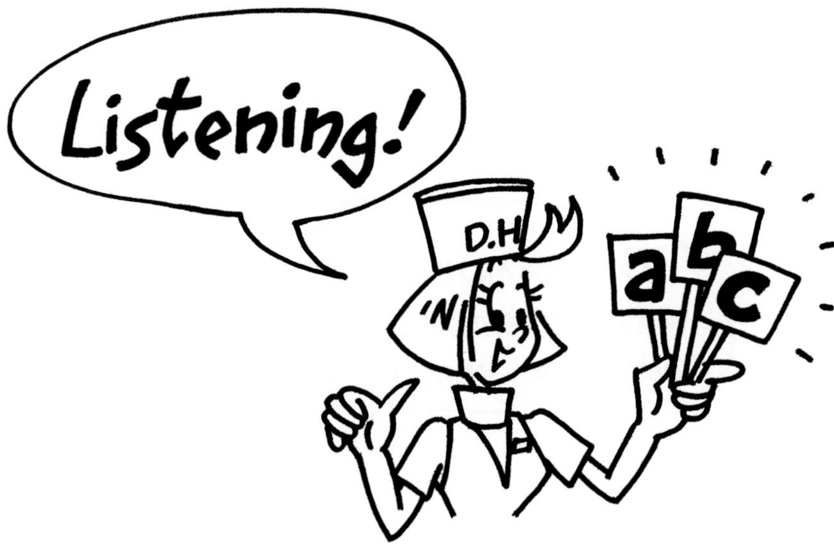

263-00488

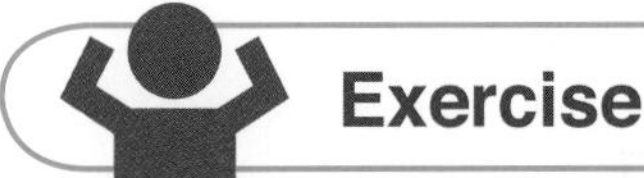

Exercise

Dialogue に出てきた表現を使って作文してみましょう.

① Is it OK to 〜？（〜してもいいですか？／大丈夫ですか？）

（例）

Is it OK to have my teeth cleaned?
（歯をきれいにしてもらっても大丈夫ですか？）
Is it OK to pay by credit card?
（クレジットカードで払ってもいいですか？）

Is it OK to ________________________________?

② There is no problem with 〜 ing.
（〜することになんら問題ありません／〜しても全くかまいません）

（例）

There is no problem with having your teeth cleaned.
（歯をきれいにすることにはなんら問題はありません）
There is no problem with working on Saturdays.
（土曜日に働くのは全くかまいません）

There is no problem with ________________________.

③ I would like to 〜 as soon as possible.
（できるだけ早く〜したいです）

（例）

I would like to make an appointment as soon as possible.
（いますぐに予約を入れたいです）
I would like to see your parents as soon as possible.
（あなたのご両親にできるだけ早くお会いしたいです）

I would like to ________________________________
as soon as possible.

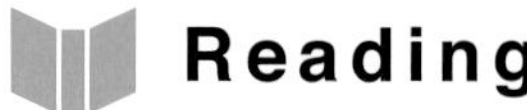

Reading

Bleeding and swollen gums during pregnancy (pregnancy gingivitis)
（妊娠中の歯肉の出血と腫脹／妊娠性歯肉炎）

Pregnancy generally worsens preexisting gum problems, sometimes dramatically. Swollen and inflamed gums which may be sore and more susceptible to bleeding are common during pregnancy. Many pregnant women show some signs of gingivitis during pregnancy. This inflammation of the gums is called pregnancy gingivitis. Gingivitis is defined as the inflammation or swelling of the gum tissues. Most cases of gingivitis are the result of poor oral hygiene. If plaque is not removed daily by brushing and flossing, the plaque can irritate the gums, making them bright red, tender, swollen, sensitive and bleed readily. During pregnancy there is a special need for good oral hygiene because pregnancy may exaggerate the body's normal response to dental plaque. Pregnancy gingivitis is influenced by the hormonal change of estrogen and progesterone which increases the blood flow to the gum tissue and causes gums to be more sensitive and vulnerable to irritation and swelling.

The hormonal changes also hinder the body's normal response to the bacteria which causes periodontal infections. This makes it easier for plaque to build up on teeth and makes more susceptible to gingivitis. It is important to note, that it is the plaque, and not the increased hormone levels that is the major cause of pregnancy gingivitis.

Swelling of the gums is usually first seen in the second month of pregnancy and generally reaches a peak by the middle of the last trimester, but it begins to decrease during the ninth month. The severity of the gingivitis can range from mild to severe depending on the gum problems existing before pregnancy. Gums usually return to normal following the delivery of a baby and the bleeding and sensitivity should diminish.

263-00488

How do you manage your bleeding and swollen gums?

Thorough oral hygiene is essential during pregnancy. You should effectively brush your teeth at least twice a day, and floss your teeth daily to remove plaque from the tooth surfaces not reached by the toothbrush. You should also visit your dental professional regularly for advice and therapy on oral disease prevention and oral health promotion while you are pregnant. This is a good time to ask your dental hygienist if you are brushing and flossing effectively and if there is room for improvement in your daily plaque control.

By practicing good oral hygiene, and visiting the dental clinic regularly, gingivitis can be prevented during pregnancy.

Here are things that you can do to prevent pregnancy gingivitis and have healthier oral hygiene:

- Visit your dentist regularly for oral checkup
- Brush at least twice a day and floss once a day
- Brush immediately after vomiting from morning sickness
- Practice good nutrition and avoid eating large amounts of refined sugar
- Rinse daily or periodically with warm salt water

Q1 Why does pregnancy gingivitis occur?

Q2 Does pregnancy gingivitis continue after the delivery of a baby?

Q3 What are the most effective methods to prevent pregnancy gingivitis?

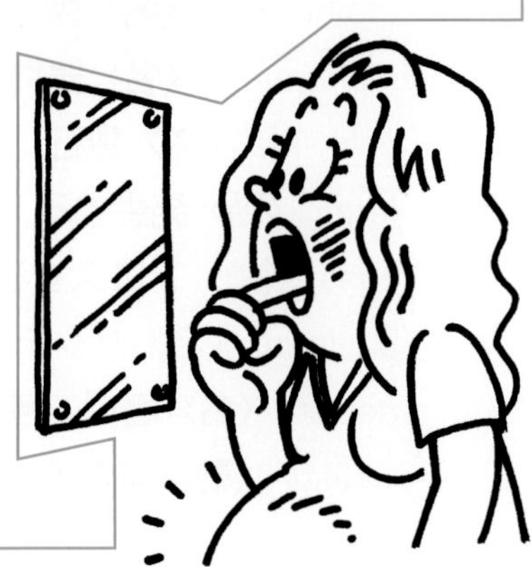

263-00488

9 Why Do I Need a Cleaning?

Warm up

One of the important roles of the dental hygienist is patient education. The patients will be much happier with their treatment and more likely to return to the clinic if they understand what is being done and the reason for the treatment.

Vocabulary

brush 〈動〉磨く
remove 〈動〉取り除く
calcium deposit 〈名〉カルシウム沈着物
plaque 〈名〉プラーク
stain 〈名〉色素性沈着物
gum line 〈名〉歯肉ライン
toothbrush 〈名〉歯ブラシ
instrument 〈名〉器具
calculus 〈名〉歯石
form 〈動〉発生する，形成する
floss 〈動〉フロスする，〈名〉フロス
bacteria 〈名〉バクテリア，細菌
debris 〈名〉歯垢，残骸
collect 〈動〉溜まる，積もる

263-00488

Dialogue

音声：09-D.mp3

Situation The dental hygienist, Ms. Yoshida, is explaining the need for cleaning to the patient, Mr. Beresford.

Mr. Beresford（B） Why do I need a cleaning? I brush my teeth every day.

Ms. Yoshida（Y） The cleaning we do removes calcium deposits, plaque and stain on the teeth and under the gum line.

B Can't my toothbrush do that?

Y I use special instruments that remove calculus and deposits that the toothbrush can't get off.

B What is calculus?

Y It is calcium deposits that form on the teeth over time. It is very hard and cannot be removed with a toothbrush.

B If you clean my teeth, is it still necessary for me to brush every day?

Y Yes. It is very important to brush and floss your teeth every day to remove plaque.

B What is plaque?

Y It is a film of bacteria and food debris that collects on the teeth and under the gum line.

B Thank you for telling me about this.

Y I will put the chair back now so that we can begin the cleaning.

B Thank you.

263-00488

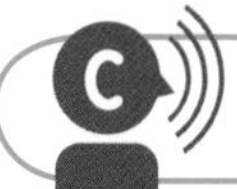

Listening 質問を聞いて，正しい答えを選びましょう

音声：09-L.mp3

1. *a* The reason for the treatment.
   b The instruments to be used in the treatment.
   c How she or he became a dental hygienist.

2. *a* Extracts a patient's teeth.
   b Bleaches a patient's teeth.
   c Removes unnecessary substance from a patient's teeth.

3. *a* Every day.
   b Every other day.
   c Every week.

4. *a* On the teeth only.
   b Under the gum line only.
   c Both on the teeth and under the gum line.

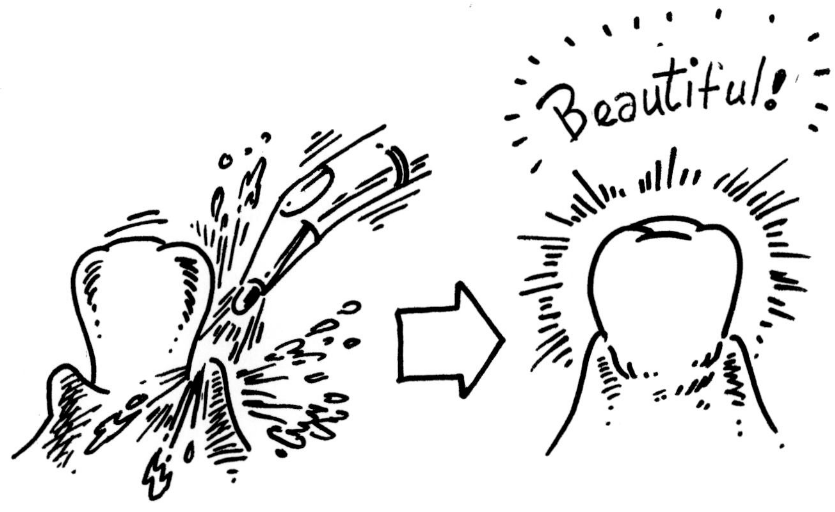

263-00488

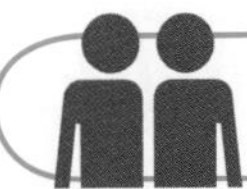

Pair Work

① まず，例にならって，患者さんからの質問に対する応答を下線部に書いてみましょう．

（例）

Patient　What is calculus?

DH　It is calcium deposits that form over time on the teeth.

Patient　What is a molar?

DH　It is ________________________________.

（例）

Patient　Is it necessary for me to brush every day?

DH　Yes. It is very important to brush your teeth every day to remove plaque.

Patient　Is it necessary for me to have a cleaning regularly?

DH　Yes. It is very important to have a cleaning regularly to ____

____.

② 次に，自分の答えとパートナーが書いた答えとを比べ，実際に音読して練習しましょう．

263-00488

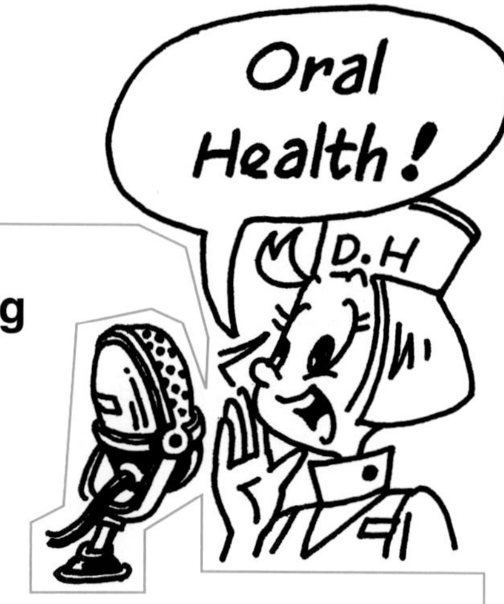

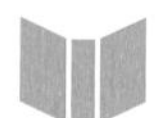

Reading

Global goals for oral health
（口腔保健に関する国際目標）

FDI (Federation of Dentaire Internationale), WHO (World Health Organization) and IADR (International Association of Dental Research) jointly proposed the global goals for oral health to be achieved by the year 2020. However there are no absolute values in the goals, as they have to be established on the basis of local situations.

Each country's situation is different not only in the epidemiology of oral diseases, but also with regard to political, socio-economic, cultural and legislative context. Therefore regional, national and local health care planners are encouraged to specify realistic goals and standards for oral health to be achieved. This is based on the spirit of the United Nations Development Program's report "Think globally, act locally".

According to the current classification of diseases and established criteria for their diagnosis, following 16 targets are listed for guidance to develop local goals.

1. Pain, 2. Functional disorder, 3. Infectious diseases, 4. Oro-pharyngeal cancer, 5. Oral manifestations of HIV infection, 6. Noma, 7. Trauma, 8. Craniofacial anomalies, 9. Dental caries, 10. Development anomalies of teeth, 11. Periodontal diseases, 12. Oral mucosal diseases, 13. Salivary gland disorders, 14. Tooth loss, 15. Health care services, 16. Health care information system.

The framework of global goals for dental caries and periodontal diseases are listed below for example.

263-00488

Dental caries

- To increase the proportion of caries free 6 -year-olds by X%.
- To reduce the DMFT particularly the D component at age 12 years by X%, with special attention to high-risk groups within population, utilizing both distributions and means
- To reduce the number of teeth extracted due to dental caries at ages 18 , 35 - 44 and 65 - 74 years by X%.

Periodontal diseases

- To reduce the number of teeth lost due to periodontal diseases by X % at ages 18 , 35 - 44 and 65 - 74 years with special reference to smoking, poor oral hygiene, stress and inter-current systemic diseases.
- To reduce the prevalence of necrotizing forms of periodontal diseases by X% by reducing exposure to risk factors such as poor nutrition, stress and immunosuppression.
- To reduce the prevalence of active periodontal infection 8 with or without loss of attachment) in all ages by X%
- To increase the proportion of people in all ages with healthy periodontium (gums and supporting bone structure) by X%.

(Reference: Global goals for oral health 2020 . International Dental Journal, 53 : 285 - 288 , 2003 .)

Q1 Why global goals do not have absolute values?
Q2 Is there a global goals for dt comportment for 6 -year-olds?
Q3 What are the risk factors of periodontal diseases?

10 Informed Consent

Part I

Warm up

It is important for the patient to understand his or her treatment before any work is done. The patient should understand the reason for the treatment, how the treatment will be done, and the cost. This is called "informed consent". In the US, the dental hygienist frequently gives this explanation because the doctor may be too busy. If the dental hygienist cannot answer the patient's questions, she should refer them to the dentist. Sometimes, the dental hygienist can draw a simple diagram of the tooth that will be treated. This will help the patient understand the procedure.

Vocabulary

frequently 〈副〉頻繁に
explanation 〈名〉説明 *cf.* explain 〈動〉説明する
refer ～ to … 〈動〉～を…に任せる
procedure 〈名〉手順，処置
root canal 〈名〉根管
gentle 〈形〉優しい，穏やかな
premolar 〈名〉小臼歯
numb 〈動〉麻痺させる
material 〈名〉材料
nerve 〈名〉神経
normally 〈副〉普通に，通常どおり

263-00488

Dialogue

音声：10_Part1-D.mp3

Situation The dental hygienist, Ms. Tatsuki, is explaining the treatment and costs to Mr. Cho, a businessman from Hong Kong.

Ms. Tatsuki（T） Hello, Mr. Cho. Dr. Matsui ① has asked me to explain the treatment plan to you. Is that OK?

Mr. Cho（C） Thank you. I would appreciate that.

T After Dr. Matsui ① examined you, he found two cavities that need treatment.

C Yes. He told me. ②

T Both are on the lower left side. ③

C Yes, and one of them hurts.

T I understand. That tooth will need root canal treatment.

C Root canal treatment? That sounds painful.

T Don't worry. Dr. Matsui ① is very gentle. ④ He will give you an anesthetic. The procedure won't be uncomfortable at all.

C Can you explain what root canal treatment is?

---

①	Dr. Nakamura	Dr. Sugiyama
②	I already heard that	He said so
③	the upper right side	the lower right side
④	nice	thoughtful

（Pair Work 参照）

263-00488

T Certainly. I will draw a picture of the tooth and show you.

C Thank you. ⑤

T Here's your tooth, right? (Ms.Tatsuki is making the drawing.) This is a premolar. It has decay, and the decay has infected the root.

C I see.

T And that is why it hurts. Dr. Matsui ⑥ will give you an anesthetic to numb the feeling in the tooth. OK?

C OK. I would appreciate that.

T Then, he will remove the infected tissue from the canal of the tooth here. (Ms. Tatsuki points to the drawing of the root.)

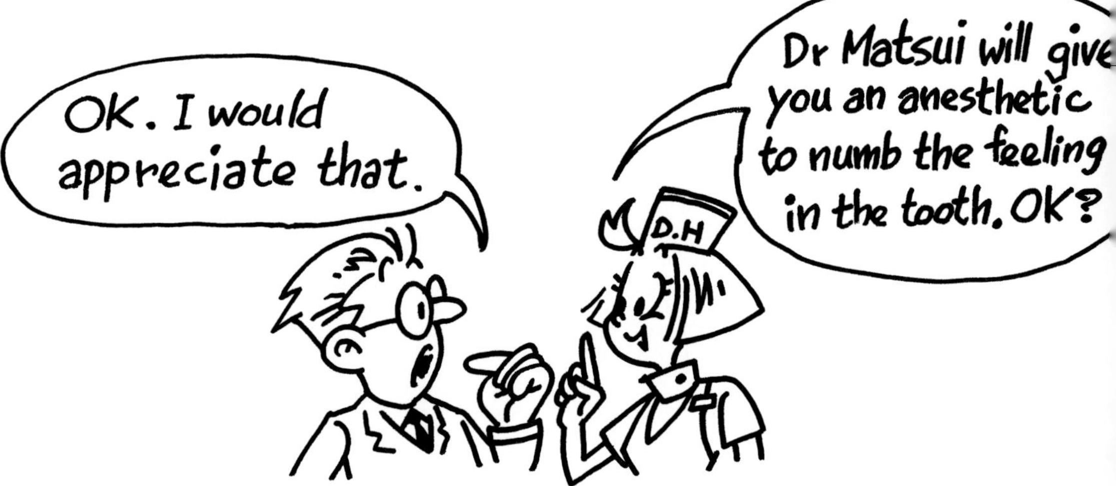

⑤ That's great	That's good
⑥ Dr. Nakamura	Dr. Sugiyama

（Pair Work 参照）

263-00488

C So the tissue will be removed?

T Yes, that's right.

C How long will that take?

T Only a few minutes. Then the doctor will put a filling material in the canal of the tooth.

C Will the tooth be dead?

T Yes. There won't be a nerve in the tooth anymore.

C Oh, no. That's not good.

T It's really not a problem. You should be able to keep the tooth and use it normally for the rest of your life.

C That is better than losing the tooth, I guess. ⑦

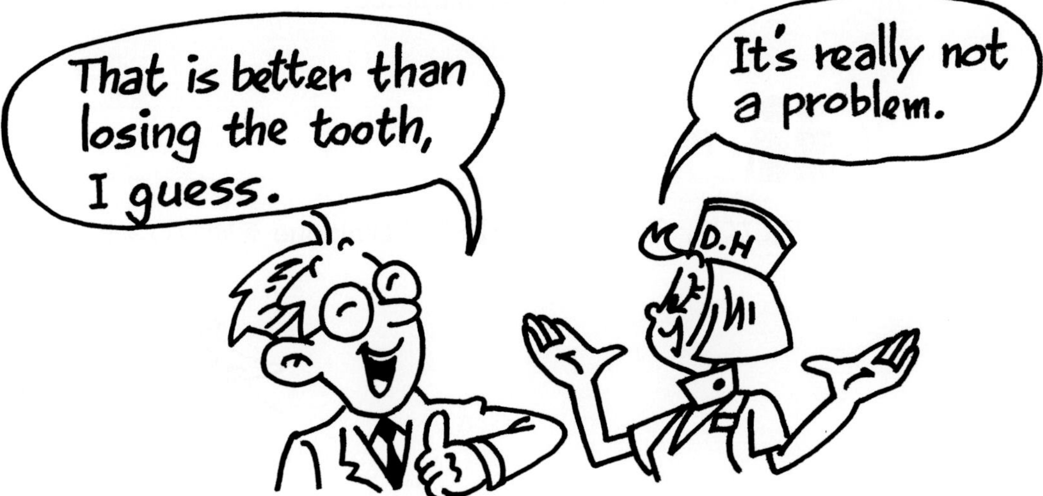

---

⑦ I'm glad to hear that　　I guess I should be satisfied with that

(Pair Work 参照)

263-00488

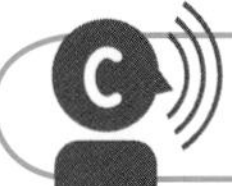

Listening 質問を聞いて，正しい答えを選びましょう

音声：10_Part1-L.mp3

1. *a* None.
   b One.
   c Two.

2. *a* Put a filling material in the tooth.
   b Remove the infected tissue from the tooth.
   c Give him an anesthetic.

3. *a* By showing an X-ray of the tooth.
   b By drawing a picture of the tooth.
   c By showing Mr. Cho's teeth with a mirror.

4. *a* It will be replaced with a new tooth.
   b It will be used normally.
   c It will be dead and extracted.

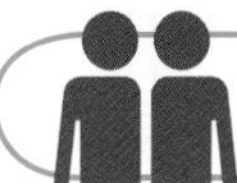

Pair Work

ペアになり，下線部を入れ替えて Dialogue を練習しましょう.

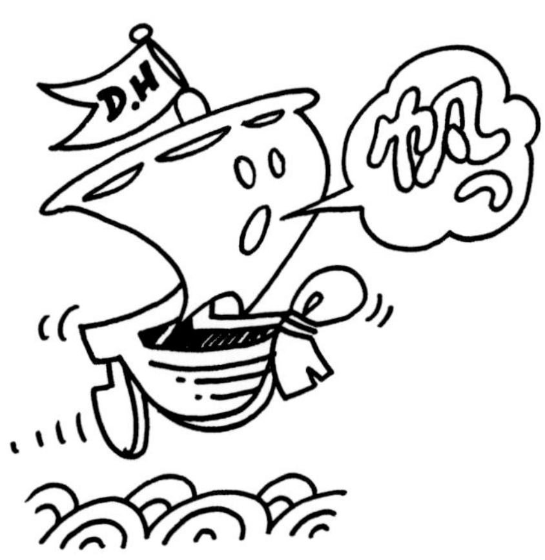

263-00488

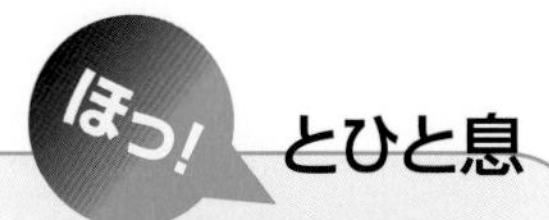

海外で活躍する歯科衛生士　4

愛知学院大学歯科衛生専門学校（現 愛知学院大学短期大学部歯科衛生学科）卒
中条さやか

●夢を追って

あなたの夢はなんですか？　具体的な夢はありますか？　歯科衛生士としてどのように働きたいですか？

私は，2001年に愛知学院大学附属歯科衛生学科を卒業しましたが，卒業後は歯科衛生士として仕事をすることもあれば，あるときは歯科助手として働かなければならないという状況で，これでいいのかなと感じ始めるようになっていました．そんなとき，ある先生に出会い，日本と米国の歯科衛生士の違いについて学んでいくうちに，米国の歯科衛生士がとても魅力的に感じるようになりました．そこで歯科衛生士学校時代にお世話になった先生に，米国で歯科衛生士をしているという足立弘美さん（p.27参照）を紹介してもらい，早速，ポートランドにある彼女の職場を見学しに行くことにしたのです．

そこには，麻酔の使用やエックス線写真撮影などを歯科衛生士の判断のもとで行うことができ，歯科衛生士も個室をもって治療にあたるという，まさに私が夢にみた光景がありました．私はすぐさま，米国で歯科衛生士を目指す決意をしました．

●理想の歯科衛生士を求めて

それからは，米国留学に向けて学校の情報収集やTOEFLの勉強を1年かけて行いました．あわせて貯金にも努めました．その結果，学生ビザを取得でき，米国のポートランドコミュニティ大学に留学することになりました．

留学後は，はじめの半年間は英語力をつけるために英語クラスを受講し，その後，歯科衛生士プログラムに進むために必須の科目（化学，数学，英語論文，人体解剖学，生理学，微生物学，栄養学）を受講するようにしました．この大学では，必須科目を終了しないと専門プログラムに参加できないのです．

歯科衛生士プログラムは非常に人気があり，前年は200人以上の応募者のなかで18人しかすすめなかったほどの難関です．でも，私は決してあきらめることはしませんでした．自分の目標に向かうために……．そして，ついに念願の歯科衛生士プログラムに進むことができました．日本とは違うことを学ぶことができ，とても刺激的です．

最近ではようやく，受け持ちの患者さんももてるようになりました．自分の患者さんのアポイントを自分でとらなくてはいけなかったり，実際に患者さんにお会いして治療を行うことは神経を使いますが，大きな喜びを感じて過ごしています．

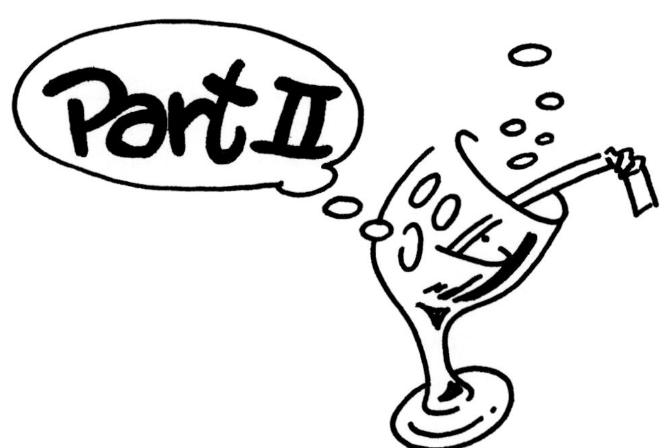

Part II

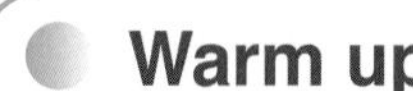

Warm up

This is a continuation of the previous dialogue.

Vocabulary

restore 〈動〉戻す，修復する
complete 〈動〉完成させる，終える
mold 〈名〉型
entire 〈形〉すべての，全体の
temporary 〈形〉仮の，一時的な
permanent 〈形〉永久の
mercury 〈名〉水銀
original 〈名〉原物

263-00488

Dialogue

音声：10_Part2-D.mp3

Situation The dental hygienist is explaining how the tooth will be restored after the root canal treatment has been completed, and how much the treatment will cost.

Mr. Cho（C） What will be done after the root treatment is completed?

Ms. Tatsuki（T） The doctor will prepare the tooth and take a mold for a crown.

C How much time will that take? ①

T The entire appointment will last about 90 minutes. Then Dr. Matsui ② will put a temporary plastic crown on the tooth.

C When do I get the permanent crown?

T It will be ready in two weeks.

C What about the other cavity?

T That one is smaller. Here, you can see it in this sketch. When you come back for the crown, he will put a filling in that tooth.

C I don't want a mercury filling.

T The doctor never uses fillings with mercury.

C That's good.

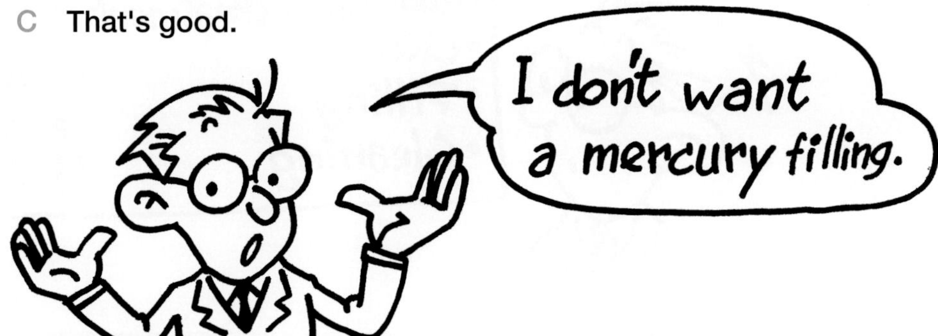
I don't want a mercury filling.

① How long will it be? How long is it going to take?
② Dr. Nakamura Dr. Sugiyama

（Pair Work 参照）

263-00488

T He will use composite resin, which is the same color as the tooth.

C That's what I want. How much does all this cost?

T The examination and X-rays today are 8,000③ yen. The root canal treatment is 30,000 yen, and the crown is 110,000 yen. I will write all of the prices here.

C That would be very helpful. ④ How much is the filling?

T That is only 20,000⑤ yen. You also should have a cleaning, which you can do today if you like. It is 8,000 yen.

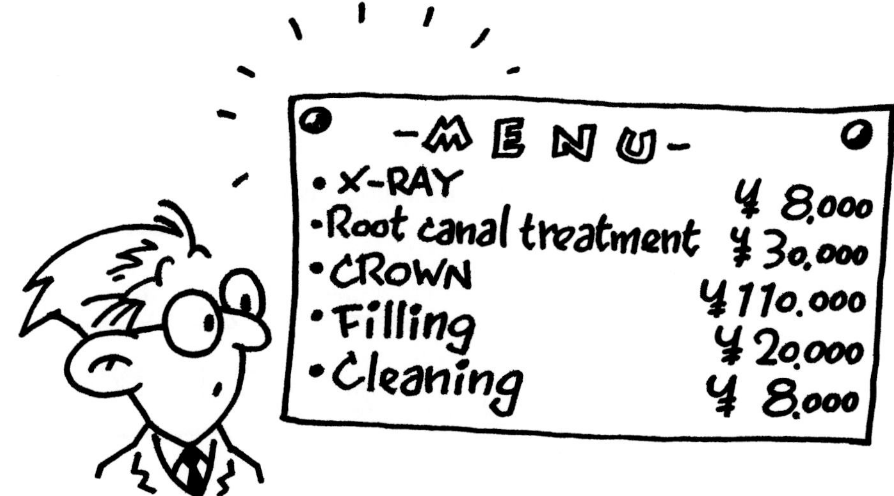
-MENU-
• X-RAY ¥ 8,000
• Root canal treatment ¥ 30,000
• CROWN ¥110,000
• Filling ¥ 20,000
• Cleaning ¥ 8,000

③ 7,000	9,000
④ appreciated	very nice
⑤ 18,000	21,000

(Pair Work 参照)

263-00488

C　I want to do that. ⑥

T　I will make a copy of this sketch for our records and then give you the original.

C　Thank you. I have to explain all this to my wife.

T　If you have any questions I can't answer, Dr. Matsui will be glad to help you.

C　Thank you.

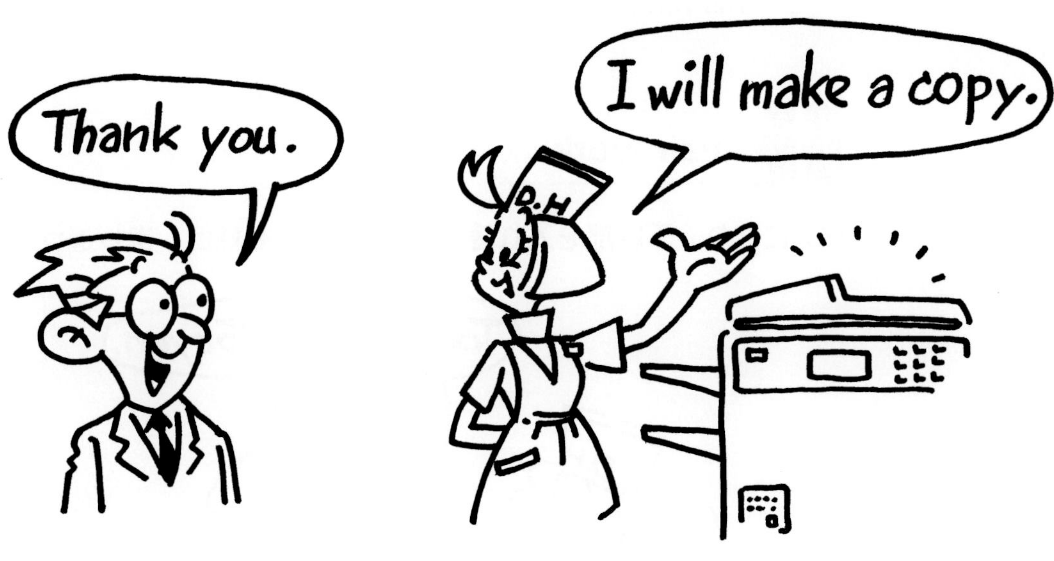

⑥ I'd like to have that　　　　I guess I should do that

（Pair Work 参照）

263-00488

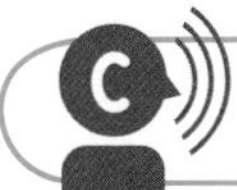

Listening 質問を聞いて，正しい答えを選びましょう

音声：10_Part2-L.mp3

1. *a* Two days.
   b Two weeks.
   c Twenty days.

2. *a* A mercury filling.
   b A plastic filling.
   c A composite resin filling.

3. *a* 8,000 yen.
   b 30,000 yen.
   c 110,000 yen.

4. *a* His boss.
   b His mother.
   c His wife.

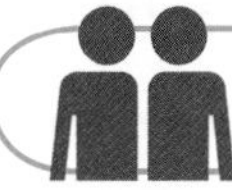

Pair Work

ペアになり，下線部を入れ替えて Dialogue を練習しましょう.

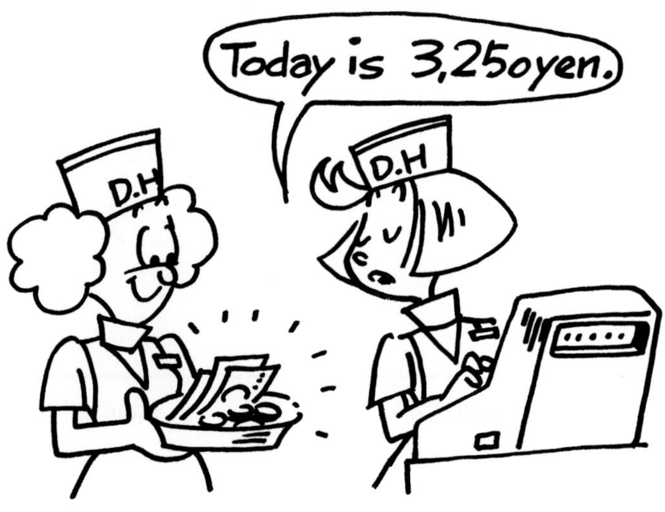

263-00488

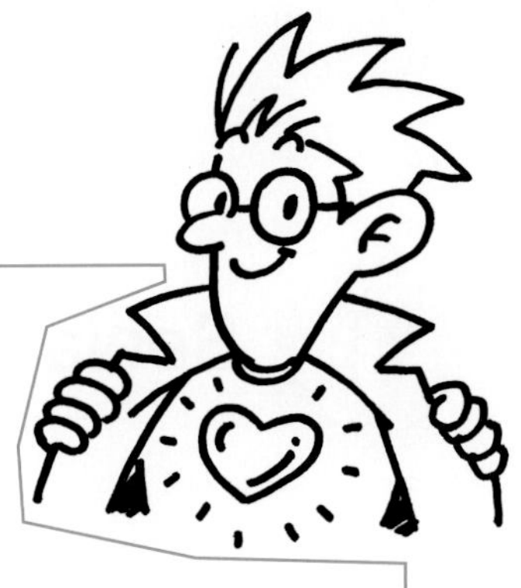

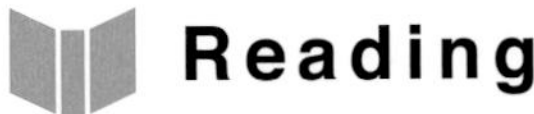

Reading

Informed consent（インフォームドコンセント）

After the Nuremberg trials, a series of trials for the prosecution Nazi Germany, from 1945 to 1946, it was generally agreed that human beings should not be experimented on without their knowledge and consent. In July, 1981 the regulations governing the requirements for informed consent of human subjects became effective in the United States.

In the medical setting, informed consent is the process by which fully informed patients can participate in choices about their health care. Health care providers give patients information about a particular treatment in order for the patients to decide whether or not they wish to undergo such procedure.

Health care providers are required by law or institutional policies to obtain informed consent before administering certain medical procedures. Although informed consent is often equated with a signed written form used to document an individual's decision, written consent is neither inherently necessary nor sufficient. Regardless of the presence or absence of documentation, informed consent requires health care providers to ensure that a patient has knowingly and voluntarily agreed to be treated. Informed consent can only be obtained after the patient has been given information about the nature of the medical procedure, its associated risks and benefits, and other alternatives.

The most important goal of informed consent is that the patients have an opportunity to be informed participants in their health care decisions. It is generally accepted that complete informed consent process includes a discussion of the following component:

1. Patient's diagnosis
2. Methods of recommended treatment / procedure
3. Possible benefits and risks of recommended treatment / procedure
4. Possible alternatives to recommended treatment / procedure
5. Possible risks of not receiving treatment / procedure
6. Possible cost of recommended treatment / procedure

Q1 What is informed consent at dental office?

Q2 Please define a list of essential components for informed consent.

Q3 Please describe the role of a dental hygienist in the consent process.

263-00488

11 Sealants

Part I

Warm up

Parents sometimes ask the dental hygienist about sealants. This is a valuable treatment and is recommended for all children who have deep grooves in their permanent molars. Of course, all explanations should be made to the child as well as to the parent. It is good to give the parent a leaflet explaining the treatment.

Vocabulary

sealant 〈名〉シーラント
valuable 〈形〉価値のある，役に立つ
recommend 〈動〉すすめる
groove 〈名〉溝
leaflet 〈名〉リーフレット，チラシ
layer 〈名〉層
molar 〈名〉大臼歯，臼歯
prevent 〈動〉防止する，避ける，予防する
decay 〈名〉齲蝕，むし歯
permanent 〈形〉永久の
X-ray 〈名〉エックス線写真

263-00488

Dialogue

音声：11_Part1-D.mp3

Situation Dr. Suzuki has recommended sealants for Bobby Miller. The dental hygienist, Ms. Kojima, is explaining why sealants are necessary to Bobby's mother.

Ms. Kojima（K） Dr. Suzuki ① said that Bobby needs sealants.

Ms. Miller（M） Why is that necessary?

K Please look at this leaflet ② while I explain.

M Thank you. ③

K A sealant is a thin layer of white plastic that is placed in the grooves of the molars to prevent decay.

M How does it help?

K The permanent molars have deep grooves where decay can easily get started.

M I didn't have sealants when I was a child. ④

K It probably would have helped you.

M Why?

K Look at your X-rays. All eight ⑤ of your molars have either a filling or a crown.

M I don't want Bobby to have teeth like mine.

① Dr. Saito	Dr. Takahashi
② picture	chart
③ OK	Sure
④ young	small
⑤ Most	Half

(Pair Work 参照)

263-00488

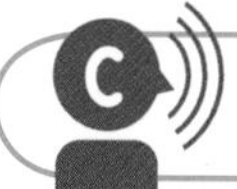

Listening 質問を聞いて，正しい答えを選びましょう

音声：11_Part1-L.mp3

1. *a* Bobby's behavior.
   b Bobby's treatment.
   c Bobby's X-rays.

2. *a* It is for the patient to prevent tooth decay.
   b It is for the doctor to examine the patient's teeth easily.
   c It is for the patient to brush his/her teeth easily.

3. *a* She thinks it's good for him to have sealants.
   b She doesn't want him to have sealants.
   c She doesn't know if it's good or bad for him.

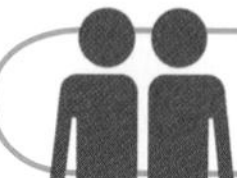

Pair Work

ペアになり，下線部を入れ替えてDialogueを練習しましょう.

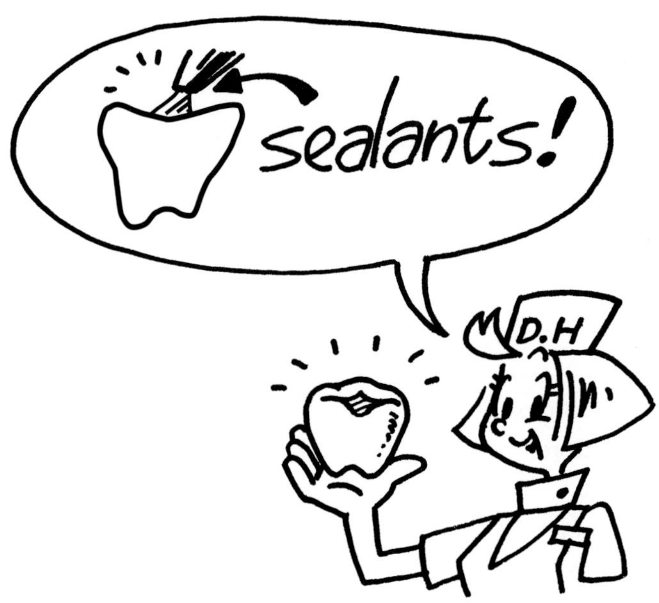

263-00488

Tooth decay often occurs on the chewing surfaces of back teeth. The good news is that sealants can offer major protection against cavities.

What causes tooth decay?

Your teeth are covered with a sticky film of bacteria, called plaque. Plaque bacteria use sugar and starch in food as a source of energy. The bacteria convert the sugar or starch into harmful acids that attack tooth enamel for as long as 20 minutes or more. Repeated attacks may cause the enamel to break down, resulting in cavities.

(ADA: SEAL OUT DECAY. より)

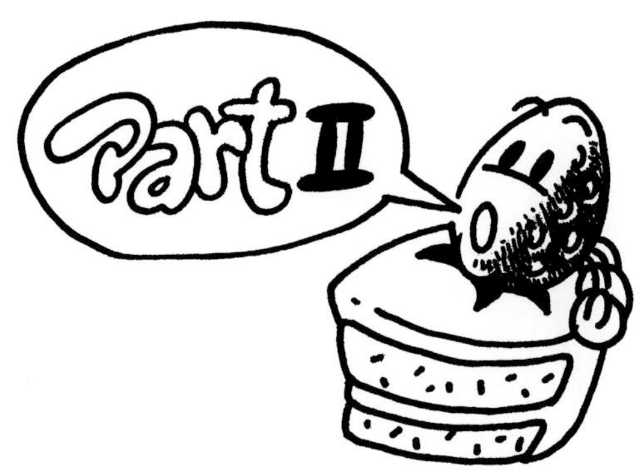

Part II

Warm up

This is a continuation of the previous dialogue. It is important to explain the treatment to children using simple words so that they will not be afraid.

Vocabulary

hurt 〈動〉痛む
uncomfortable 〈形〉不快な
pretend 〈動〉～のふりをする
fingernail 〈名〉（手の）指の爪
toothpaste 〈名〉歯磨剤，歯磨き粉
electric brush 〈名〉電動ブラシ
tickle 〈動〉くすぐったい，こそばゆい
wash off 〈動〉洗い流す
vacuum cleaner 〈名〉掃除機
liquid plastic 〈名〉液状プラスチック
scrape off 〈動〉削り落とす

263-00488

Dialogue

音声：11_Part2-D.mp3

Situation Ms. Kojima is explaining to the patient Bobby how the sealants will be done.

Bobby（B） Is the sealant difficult to do?

Ms. Kojima（K） It is very easy. I will show you what Dr. Suzuki ① will do.

B Does it hurt?

K No. It's not uncomfortable ② at all. Please give me your hand and I will show you how it is done.

B OK.

K We will pretend to do a sealant on your fingernail.

B That sounds like fun. ③

K Dr. Suzuki ① will put toothpaste on the electric brush and clean your tooth like this.

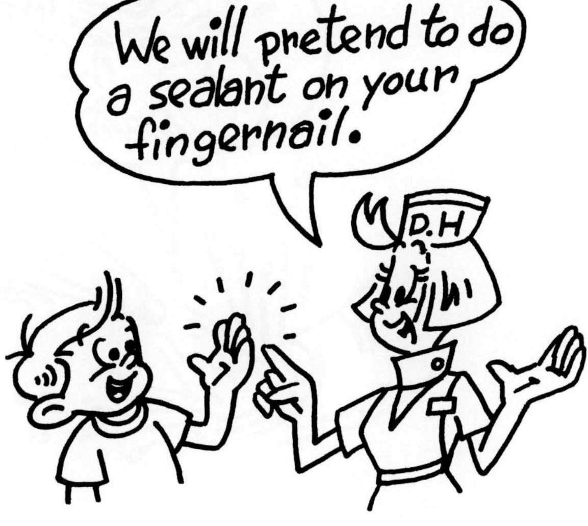

① Dr. Saito	Dr. Takahashi
② disturbing	painful
③ I see	That sounds interesting

（Pair Work 参照）

263-00488

B That tickles.

K Next he will wash off ④ the toothpaste with a spray of water like this.

B What is that thing that looks like a vacuum cleaner in your hand?

K This is a vacuum cleaner for your mouth. I will use it to clean the water that I spray on your fingernail.

B This is fun. ⑤

K Then I will put this white liquid plastic on your fingernail, just like Dr. Suzuki ⑥ will put it on your tooth.

B Cool.

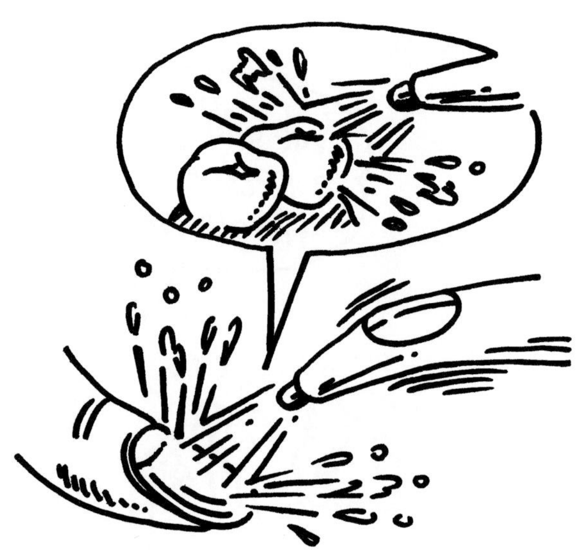

---

④ remove	rinse off
⑤ Interesting	I like it
⑥ Dr. Saito	Dr. Takahashi

(Pair Work 参照)

263-00488

K Next I will put a light on the plastic for a few seconds. The light makes the plastic hard.

B Wow. It looks like a contact lens.

K You can easily scrape this off of your fingernail. But when Dr. Suzuki ⑦ puts it on your tooth it will stay on for many years.

B Great. ⑧

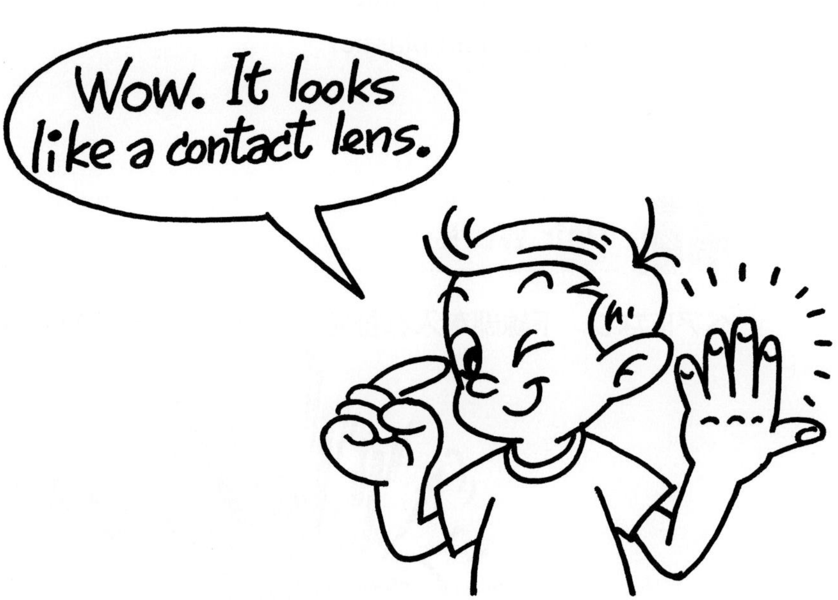

⑦ Dr. Saito	Dr. Takahashi
⑧ Wonderful	Excellent

（Pair Work 参照）

263-00488

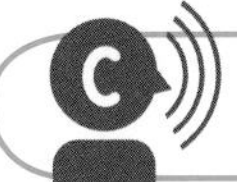

Listening 質問を聞いて，正しい答えを選びましょう

音声：11_Part2-L.mp3

1. *a* Showed him how to use an electric toothbrush.
   b Explained to him about the treatment procedure.
   c Put toothpaste on his fingernail.

2. *a* He enjoyed it.
   b He was scared by it.
   c He didn't like it.

3. *a* Explain the treatment procedure.
   b Put liquid plastic.
   c Examine the teeth.

4. *a* Gets rid of liquid plastic.
   b Softens liquid plastic.
   c Hardens liquid plastic.

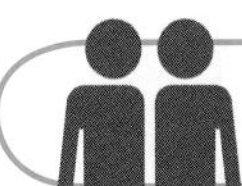

Pair Work

ペアになり，下線部を入れ替えて Dialogue を練習しましょう．

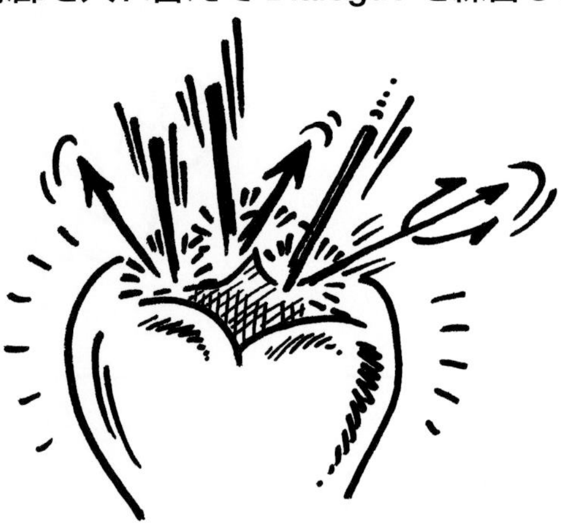

263-00488

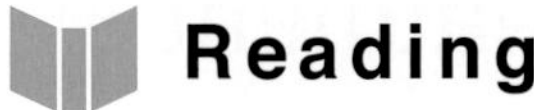

Reading

Why Sealants?（シーラントとは？）

Sealants are a thin layer of plastic that is bonded onto the chewing surface of the back teeth to prevent decay. They are especially appropriate for the six-year molars and twelve-year molars as these teeth are the most likely to get decay. Teeth have small grooves and fissures that are very difficult to clean, even with diligent brushing. When plastic is placed in these grooves, decay can be prevented by closing up the space where bacteria and food can get in and cause decay. The procedure is very simple, takes only a few minutes and does not require anesthetic or any cutting of the tooth. The surface of the tooth is first cleaned and a small amount of liquid plastic material is flowed into the grooves. A light is then placed over the plastic for a few seconds, causing it to harden. The sealants will generally last between two to ten years, and will probably have to be replaced once or twice before your child reaches adulthood. Your dentist will check that the sealants are tight each time your child comes in for a checkup, and replace or repair any places that have chipped out.

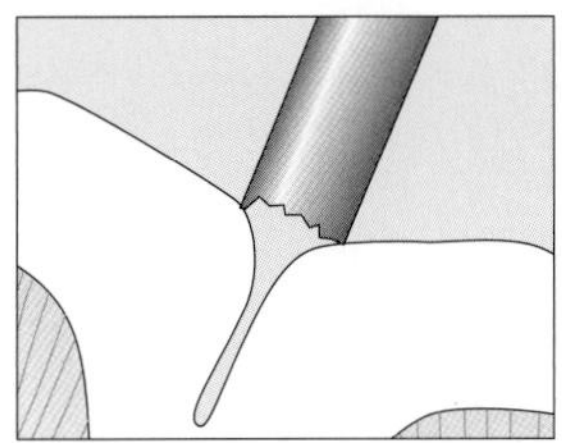

The fissure in this molar is so small that even a toothbrush bristle cannot clean it.

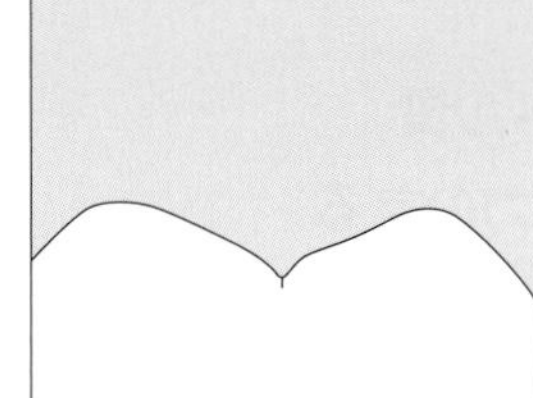

This shows a typical chewing surface of a permanent molar.

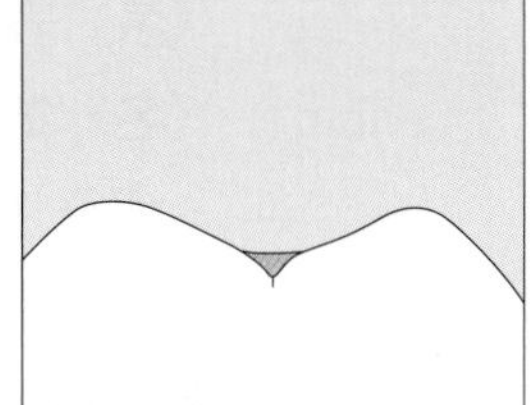

After placement of the sealant, food and bacteria are effectively blocked from getting into the grooves.

263-00488

12 Fluoride Treatment

Warm up

Before doing dental treatment on a child, the parent must be informed what is being done and why. This should be done for fillings, extractions and even fluoride treatment.

Vocabulary

fluoride 〈名〉フッ素
thoroughly 〈副〉しっかりと，完全に
solution 〈名〉溶液
concentration 〈名〉濃度，集中
ion 〈名〉イオン
seep 〈動〉浸透する
surface 〈名〉表面
enamel 〈名〉エナメル質
resistant 〈形〉抵抗力のある
effective 〈形〉効果的な
tablet 〈名〉錠剤
incorporate 〈動〉結合させる，混ぜる
jaw 〈名〉顎

263-00488

Dialogue

音声：12-D.mp3

Situation The dental hygienist, Ms. Nonaka, is explaining to Ms. Woods why fluoride treatment is necessary for her son's teeth.

Ms. Woods（W） What is fluoride treatment?

Ms. Nonaka（N） After thoroughly cleaning your child's teeth I will put a soft plastic tray with a solution of high concentration fluoride in his mouth for four minutes.

W Why do you do this?

N The fluoride ions seep into the outer surface of the teeth and make the enamel resistant to decay.

W But I brush his teeth with fluoride toothpaste. Isn't that enough?

N It is important to use fluoride toothpaste, especially for children.

W So why do you do the fluoride treatment here?

N The treatment we do here uses a high concentration of fluoride. It is more effective than the fluoride in toothpaste.

W I give my child fluoride tablets every day. Is the fluoride treatment still necessary?

N Fluoride tablets are very good for his teeth, but the fluoride treatment here is still necessary. The two are different.

W How is that?

N The fluoride in the tablets you give him are incorporated into the teeth as they develop in the jaw.

W How is that different from the fluoride treatment done here?

263-00488

N The treatment we do gets the fluoride ion into the surface layer of the enamel of the teeth that have already appeared.

W How often should the fluoride treatment be done?

N It should be done every six months when you bring him here for his regular examination.

W Thank you for explaining everything to me.

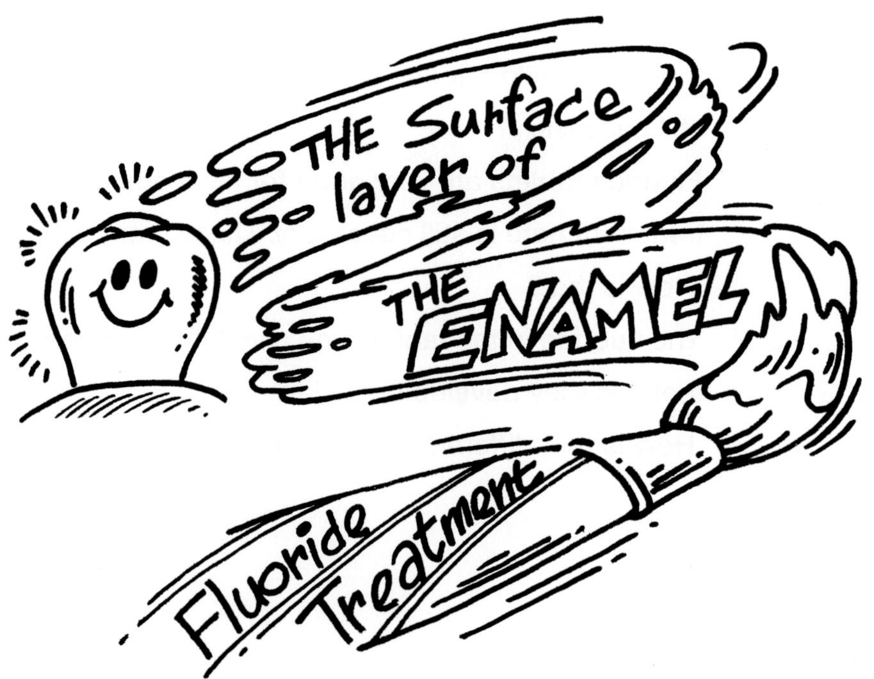

263-00488

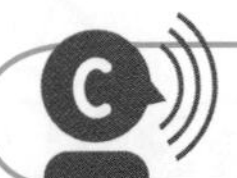

Listening 質問を聞いて，正しい答えを選びましょう

音声：12-L.mp3

1. *a* Four minutes.
   b Fourteen minutes.
   c Forty seconds.

2. *a* Help the teeth grow faster.
   b Make the teeth whiter.
   c Make the teeth stronger.

3. *a* Because they are effective against different parts of teeth.
   b Because his mother is sometimes too busy to give it to him.
   c Because he doesn't like to take fluoride tablets every day.

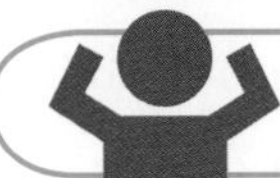

Exercise

Dialogue を読み返し，“Fluoride tablet” と歯科医院で行う “Fluoride treatment”とは何か，その違いがわかるように日本語で説明しましょう.

Fluoride tablet とは……

Fluoride treatment とは……

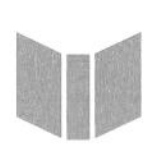

Reading

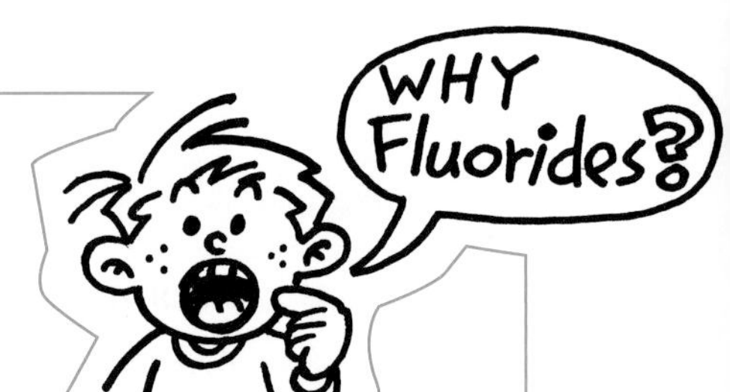

Fluoride: How does it work?（フッ化物の働き）

Fluoride is a completely natural substance that can be found in many things, like the water we drink and the food we eat. Decades ago, scientific research found that children who lived in places where fluoride occurred naturally in the water, had fewer dental cavities. Fluoride is the most powerful agent available today to fight tooth decay.

Fluoride that is absorbed by your body is used by the enamel-forming cells that build your teeth to make stronger enamel. Fluoride works whether it is swallowed or applied to the teeth, but direct contact with the teeth is especially important.

Topical fluoride - fluoride that is directly applied to the outside of the enamel either at a dentist's office or through at-home use of a topical fluoride, such as a fluoride toothpaste or mouthrinse - makes the crystals that form enamel more durable.

Tooth enamel crystals that have fluoride are much more resistant to attack by the bacterial acids that cause tooth decay. They are less likely to breakdown and cause the tooth surface to become porous. Fluoride also acts with minerals in saliva to heal small spots of decay before they develop into holes which would need filling.

Fluoride is used in many forms worldwide: fluoridated water, foods (fluoridated salt and milk), fluoride supplements (tablet or liquid), direct fluoride applications to the teeth, and fluoride toothpastes. While it cannot prevent all decay, it can provide a very high level of protection. The amounts of fluoride recommended by dentists are harmless and cause no ill effects at all.

Q1 Is fluoride a natural element?

Q2 Please describe three kinds of topical fluoride application methods.

Q3 Please describe three kinds of systemic fluoride application methods.

263-00488

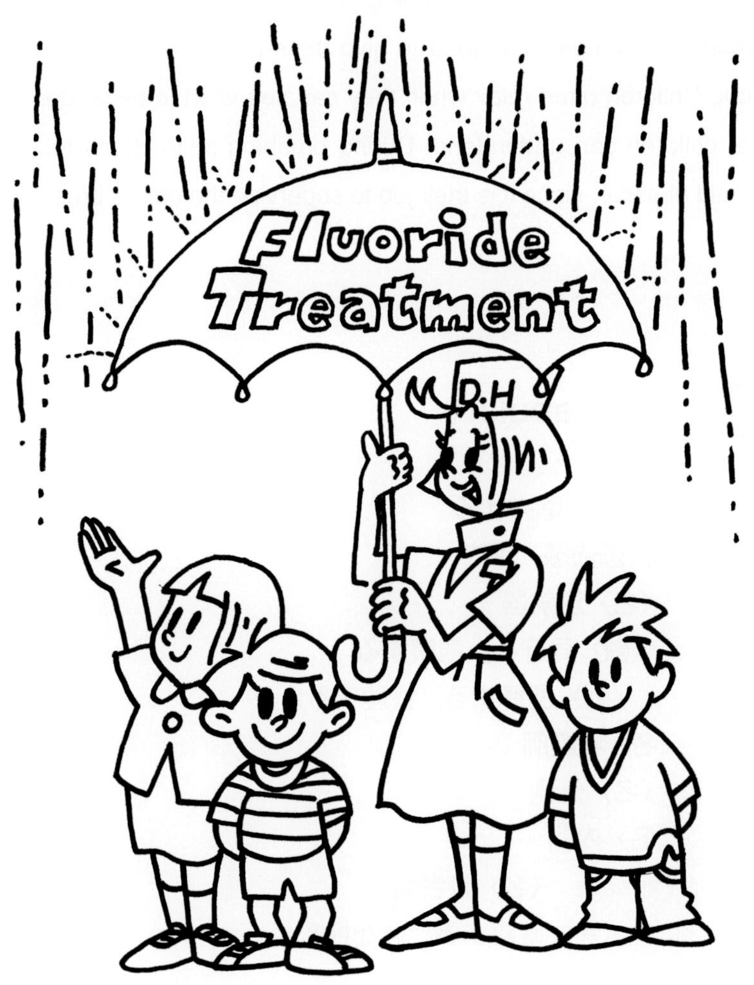

263-00488

13 Tooth Brushing Instructions for a Child

Warm up

One of the important roles of the dental hygienist in treating children is to eliminate any fear they might have about the dentist. When cleaning younger children's teeth, explain everything you do and show them all of the instruments, except the syringe. It is good to give them a mirror so they can watch when you work. Children often relax when they can see what is being done. Use only words that children can understand. During brushing instructions for a child the parent should observe, since it is their job to supervise the child's brushing every day.

Vocabulary

eliminate 〈動〉除去する
fear 〈名〉恐怖感，不安
syringe 〈名〉注射器
observe 〈動〉見守る，観察する
supervise 〈動〉監督する，管理する
nurse 〈名〉看護師
outside 〈名〉外側
inside 〈名〉内側
chewing surface 〈名〉咬合面
make sure 〈熟〉確認する，念を押す

263-00488

Dialogue

音声：13-D.mp3

Situation The dental hygienist, Ms. Taniguchi, is giving tooth brushing instructions to Janie, who is seven years old.

Janie (J) Who are you?

Ms. Taniguchi (T) I am a dental nurse. ①

J What are you going to do to me?

T I want to show you how to clean your teeth.

J Is it going to hurt?

T Of course not. ② Please look at the mirror.

J OK. ③

T First brush the outside of the teeth like this. Please try it yourself.

J OK. Is this good? ④

T That's fine. ⑤ Now go all the way around the outside of the teeth, brushing each tooth ten times like this.

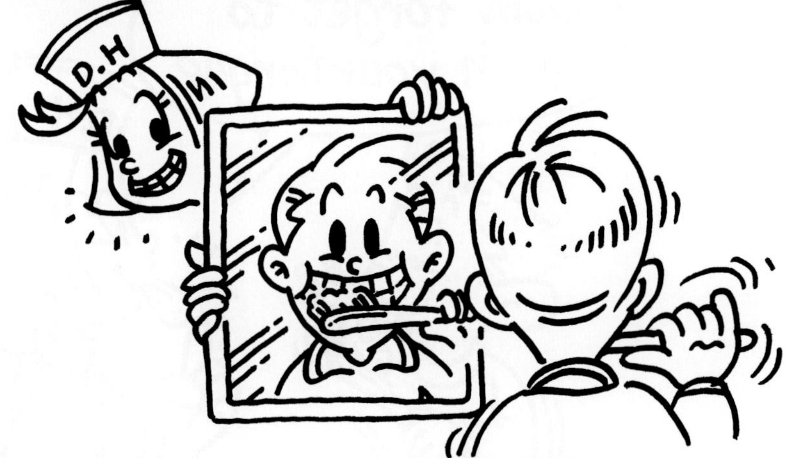

① (Your name)	(Your name)
② No, not at all	Don't worry
③ Sure	Alright
④ How am I doing?	Like this?
⑤ You're doing great!	That's great!

(Pair Work 参照)

263-00488

J　This tickles.

T　Then brush the inside of the teeth the same way.

J　This is fun. ⑥

T　Now brush the chewing surface.

J　I enjoy this.

T　Then do all the top teeth the same way, and don't forget to brush your tongue.

J　OK.

T　Your mother should help you to make sure all of your teeth are clean.

J　She helps me every day. ⑦

T　That's good. ⑧ And after brushing, your mother will floss all of your teeth.

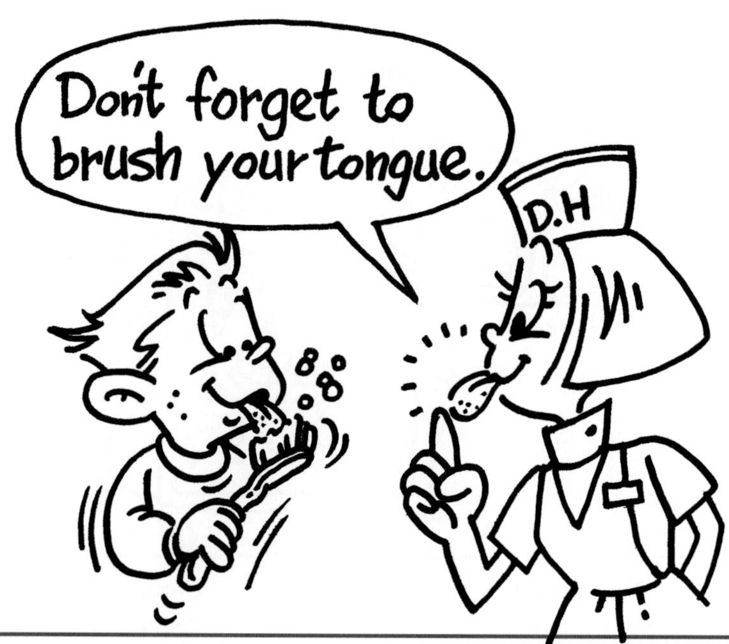

⑥ I like this	This is very interesting
⑦ She's always helpful	She always assists me
⑧ That's great	That's nice

（Pair Work 参照）

263-00488

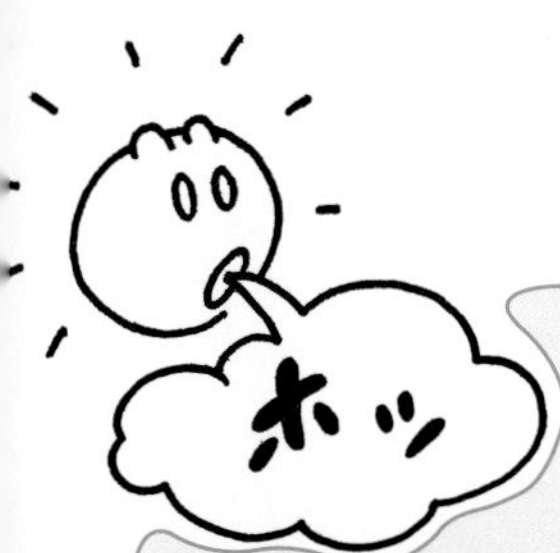

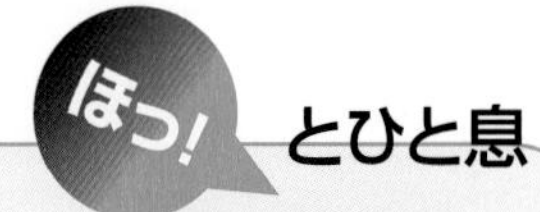

海外で活躍する歯科衛生士　5

日本歯科大学附属歯科専門学校歯科衛生士科（現 日本歯科大学東京短期大学歯科衛生学科）卒
藤山美里

●カンボジアでの歯科保健活動へ

私は歯科衛生士学校卒業後に就職した会社でおもに学校歯科保健活動に携わりました．個人差などはあるものの，子どもたちの口腔内状態は比較的上昇傾向にあるなと実感しながら仕事をしていたところ，カンボジアで歯科保健活動をしている「NPOカムカムクメール」と出会う機会に恵まれました．そこで「カンボジアの子どもたちには歯を磨く習慣が定着していなく，むし歯がとても多い」という日本とは正反対の状態を聞き，また，教科書でしか見たことのないようなひどい状態の口腔内写真を見て，とても衝撃的であったと同時に非常に興味深く思いました．そして，「いままでの経験を活かしてカンボジアの現状をよくしたい！」という思いがたんだん強くなり，会社を退職してカンボジアでの活動に参加することにしました．

●歯科衛生士もできる国際貢献

カンボジアは，長年の内戦の影響により歯科に関する知識の普及がいまだに遅れています．そこで「NPOカムカムクメール」では，治療ではなく予防に重点を置いた健康教育を現地の人々と協力しながら行っています．生活習慣を変えることや口腔内状態を良好にすることは非常に時間がかかることです．将来的にはカンボジア人の手だけでよりよくしていってほしいというのが理想なので，その日がくるまでこの活動に携わっていきたいと思っています．

このコラムを通じて私が皆さんに知っていただきたいことは「歯科衛生士も国際協力ができる！」ということです．私は現在，母校の非常勤講師もしていますが，担当している国際歯科医療援助論の講義では「国際協力をしよう！」というテーマで学生一人ひとりに簡単な手作り絵本を作成してもらっています．それを現地の子どもたちに届けるとみんな大喜びで，こちらも幸せな気持ちになれます．

いつの日かカンボジアの子どもたちの素敵な笑顔からむし歯がなくなることを夢みて，これからも活動を続けていきたいと思います．

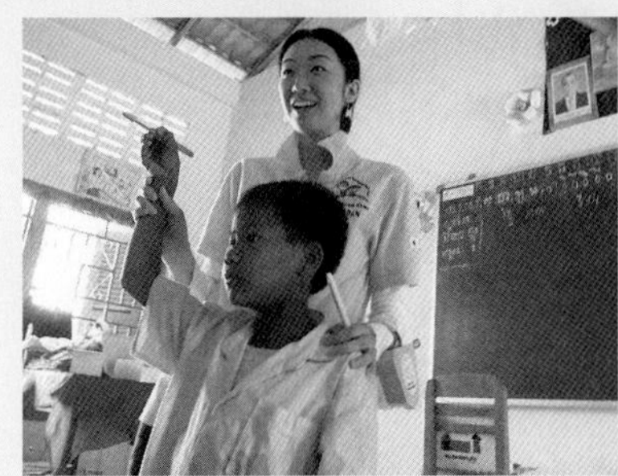
小学校での歯磨き指導

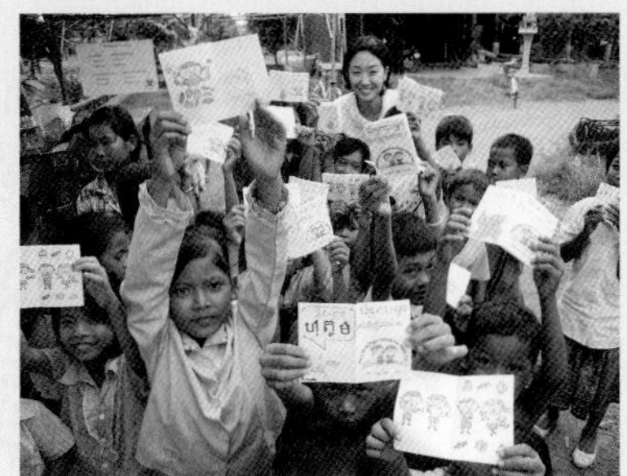
絵本を手に喜ぶ子どもたち

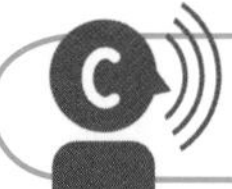

Listening 質問を聞いて，正しい答えを選びましょう

音声：13-L.mp3

1. *a* Happy.
   b Sad.
   c Worried.

2. *a* The outside.
   b The inside.
   c The chewing surfaces.

3. *a* Brushing the tongue.
   b Brushing outside of the teeth.
   c Brushing the chewing surfaces.

4. *a* She will do it herself.
   b Her mother.
   c Ms. Taniguchi.

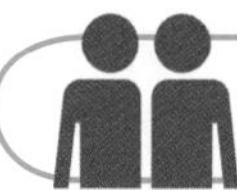

Pair Work

ペアになり，下線部を入れ替えて Dialogue を練習しましょう．

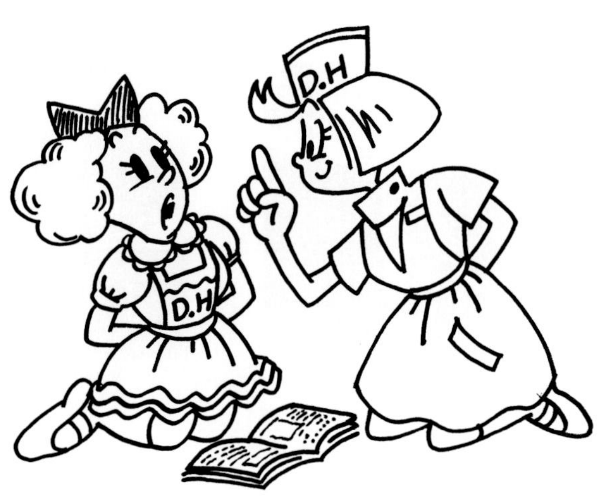

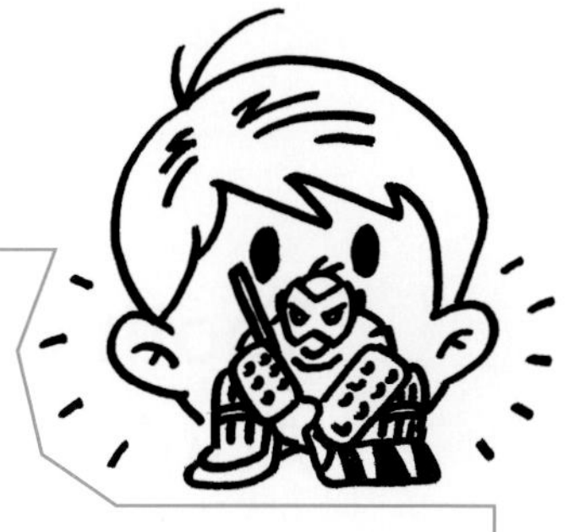

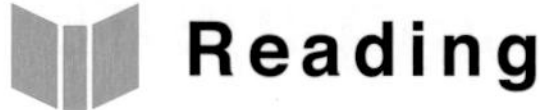

Reading

Care for child's teeth（子どもの歯のケア）

The baby teeth start to develop at about 6 months of age and this will be completed by 2 and a half years. Children will get all 20 of these baby teeth by this age. At 6 years they will start to get their adult teeth. By 12 years of age they will have all their adult teeth - 28 in total.

Here are helpful hints for healthy teeth:

- Wipe baby's gums with a clean, moist cloth after each feed. Start cleaning teeth as soon as they appear in the mouth. Use a small, soft toothbrush in the morning and evening, remembering to brush around the gum margins, and biting surfaces of all teeth. The easiest way to brush a child's teeth is from behind. Raise the chin, rest the head against you so you can see over it and down in to the mouth.
- Up to the age of about 8 or 9 years, you should help their children brush their teeth at least once a day. Always have an adult supervise while tooth brushing.
- Use only a pea-sized amount of low fluoride toothpaste or a smear of regular strength fluoride toothpaste for children over one year old. Avoid toothpastes that are brightly colored or contain attractive flavoring agents so that children do not think toothpaste is for eating. Ask young children to spit out the toothpaste and rinse after brushing.
- Begin flossing your children's teeth when the teeth begin to fit closely together. By the age of 13 they should be able to floss by themselves.
- Supervise the use of the feeding bottle to avoid nursing caries. This form of tooth decay can be caused by giving a bottle containing liquids such as fruit juice, milk or sweetened liquids at bedtime or for long periods during the day. If an infant needs a bottle to go to sleep or as a comforter, then plain water should be given in the bottle.
- Give a variety of healthy foods and snacks such as fruit, vegetable, bread, pasta and cereals. Water and plain milk should be the usual drink. Cut down the number of in-between meal sugary snacks and drinks, as they may increase the risk of tooth decay.
- Regular dental check-up should start at about 1 to 2 years of age. Dental professionals can advise you on diet, toothbrushing and the use of fluoride.

Q1　Do parents have to help their young child's tooth brushing?
Q2　Why is bottle feeding at night not so good?
Q3　What is recommended for child's between meals?

14 Tooth Brushing Instructions for an Adult

Warm up

When giving brushing instructions to the patient, it is important that she has a mirror to see what is being done. She must understand how and why she has to brush her teeth.

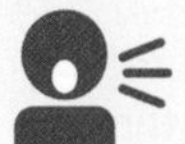

Vocabulary

instruction 〈名〉指導
exchange student 〈名〉交換留学生
regularly 〈副〉規則的に，定期的に
cause 〈動〉引き起こす
disease 〈名〉病気，疾病
breath 〈名〉息，呼吸
adequate 〈形〉十分な
sticky 〈形〉粘着性のある，なかなか取れない
properly 〈副〉正しく，適切に ***cf.*** proper 〈形〉正しい，適切な
aim 〈動〉ねらいを定める
bristle 〈名〉（ブラシなどの）毛
injure 〈動〉傷つける，痛める
circular motion 〈名〉円を描くような動き
outer 〈形〉外側の ***cf.*** inner 〈形〉内側の
chewing surface 〈名〉咬合面
quit 〈動〉やめる
accumulate 〈動〉蓄積する，増大する

263-00488

Dialogue

音声：14-D.mp3

Situation The dental hygienist, Ms. Matsuda, is giving brushing instructions to Ms. Cohen, who is an exchange student in Gotemba.

Ms. Cohen（C） Is it really necessary to brush my teeth three times every day?

Ms. Matsuda（M） Plaque collects on the teeth in only a few hours. If the plaque is not removed regularly it can cause tooth decay, gum disease and bad breath.

C But I use mouthwash. Isn't that enough?

M No. Mouthwash alone is not adequate. Brushing removes the sticky plaque on the surfaces of the teeth and floss removes it from between the teeth.

C Could you please show me how to brush properly?

M Certainly. First hold this mirror and watch while I show you.

C OK.

M Aim the bristles of the brush at a 45 degree angle with the teeth, like this.

C Doesn't that hurt the gums?

M No, not if you use the right type of brush, and the proper technique. You should use a toothbrush with bristles soft enough not to injure the gums.

C I understand.

M Brush two or three teeth at a time with a circular motion. Then move the brush forward like this and brush two or three more.

263-00488

C This is going to take a long time.

M Not so long. You should take about three minutes to brush all of your teeth.

C That's not so bad.

M After you have brushed the outer surfaces of the teeth, brush the inner surfaces, which are next to the tongue.

C I never did that before.

M That's why you have so much plaque on your teeth. Finally, brush the chewing surfaces of the teeth.

C Is that all?

M No. Not yet. You have to do the upper teeth the same way.

C Then can I quit?

M There is one more thing. You should also brush the tongue.

C Why? I never did that before.

M Bacteria that accumulate on the tongue can cause bad breath.

C Well, I certainly don't want that.

M You should brush your teeth three times each day and floss all of them at least once every day.

C Wow. I will have the cleanest teeth in town.

M I hope so.

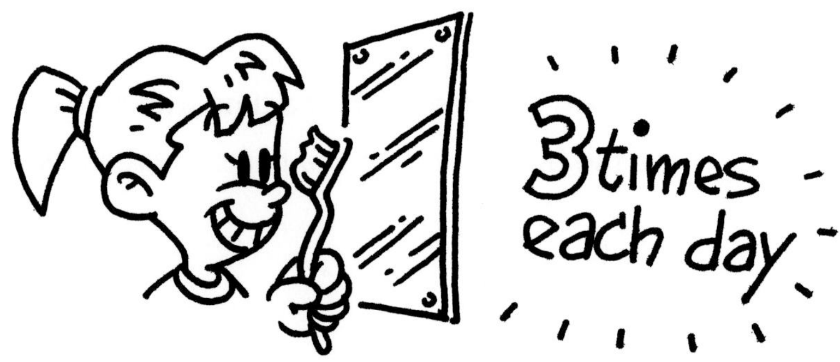

263-00488

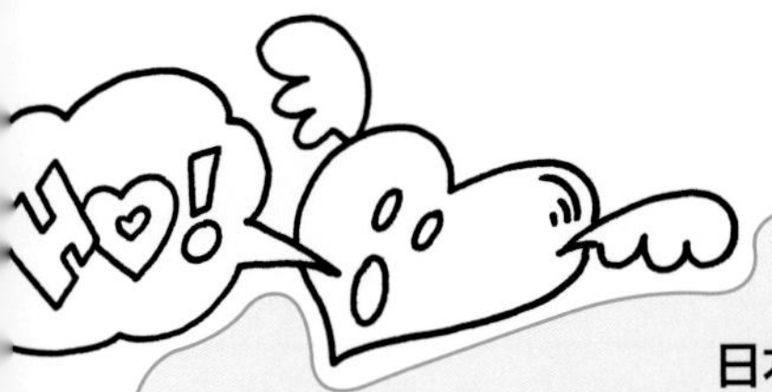

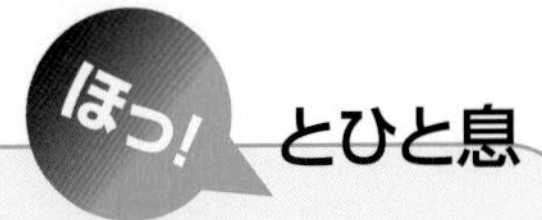

日本歯科衛生学会と国際歯科衛生士連盟

元 日本大学歯学部附属歯科衛生専門学校
柳沢嘉江

日本では2006年に日本歯科衛生学会が設立され，同年11月には東京国際フォーラムで第1回学術大会が開催されました．「歯科衛生士業務の向上を目指して—これからの臨床教育を考える—」「高齢社会の健康とQOLを支える歯科衛生士の役割」という2つの記念シンポジウムや一般会員からのたくさんの研究発表が行われ，会員の熱い息遣いを感じる学会が大盛況のなかで幕を閉じました．

日本には現在約8万人の就業歯科衛生士が存在し，歯科診療所をはじめ病院，保健施設，保健所，保健センターなどで活躍しています．業務は，日常的なことから専門化された高度なものまで，対象も胎児から寝たきりの人あるいは全身疾患をもっている高齢者までと，広い範囲に及んでいます．こうした活動のなかから，歯科衛生士の視点で社会のニーズを知り，さらに問題点を発見し，科学的根拠を見い出していく，そしてそのための調査や実験を行い，その結果を発表して多くの人の意見を聞いたり日々の活動に活かしていく，このことは歯科衛生士の業務を充実させるために不可欠なことです．日本歯科衛生学会は，歯科衛生士の活動を推進するための研究発表の場として，また学会雑誌発行などの学術研究のための機関として，日本歯科衛生士会により設立されたものです．日本歯科衛生士会の学生部員は同時に日本歯科衛生学会の学生会員となるので，学生のうちから学術大会へ積極的に参加し，さらに発表や学術誌への投稿などに意欲的に挑戦してほしいと思います．

一方，国際歯科衛生士連盟（IFDH：International Federation of Dental Hygienists）は1986年に公式に発足したもので，国際歯科連盟（FDI）および国際保健機構（WHO）と連携をとりながら世界の口腔衛生の問題に対応しています．IFDHは各国を代表する歯科衛生士会で構成され，現在25ヵ国が加盟しています（p.125参照）．3年に一度，各国のもち回りでシンポジウムが開催され，日本でも1975年と1995年に東京で行われました．シンポジウムには，各国から予防またはケアの技術，最新の研究結果などが多数提出され，日本の会員からも毎回数題が発表されています．開会式，閉会式，Welcome Receptionや社交行事では楽しい企画が組まれ，華やかな民族衣装がみられたり，参加者のお国訛りの英語によるにぎやかなおしゃべりで国際交流の輪が広がります．こちらにも是非参加してほしいと思います．なお，IFDHは学術誌International Journal of Dental Hygieneを年4回発行しています．

IFDH各国代表者会議（日本歯科衛生士会・松田智子先生提供）

参考文献・資料

1）社団法人日本歯科衛生士会ガイドブック．日本歯科衛生士会，2006，8〜9.
2）武井典子：学会設立の目指すもの．日本歯科衛生学会雑誌，1（1）：9，2006.
3）日本口腔衛生学会歯科衛生士委員会：歯科衛生士の学会活動と専門性の推進を考える．デンタル ハイジーン，25（2）：173〜175，2005.

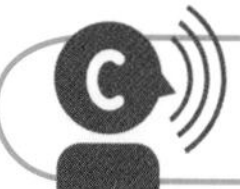

Listening 質問を聞いて，正しい答えを選びましょう

音声：14-L.mp3

1. *a* In a few minutes.
   b In a few hours.
   c In a few days.

2. *a* To hold a mirror.
   b To aim the toothbrush at a 45 degree angle.
   c To floss her teeth.

3. *a* Because they are less expensive.
   b Because they are harmless to the gums.
   c Because they are easier to use.

4. *a* To prevent tooth decay.
   b To prevent bad breath.
   c To prevent plaque.

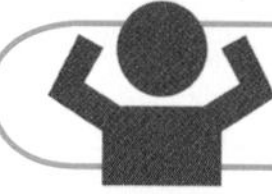

Exercise

Dialogue を読み返し，Ms. Matsuda が行った歯磨き指導を順に日本語で説明しなさい.

1. 手鏡を患者さんに渡す.
2.
3.
4.
5.
6.
7.
8.

263-00488

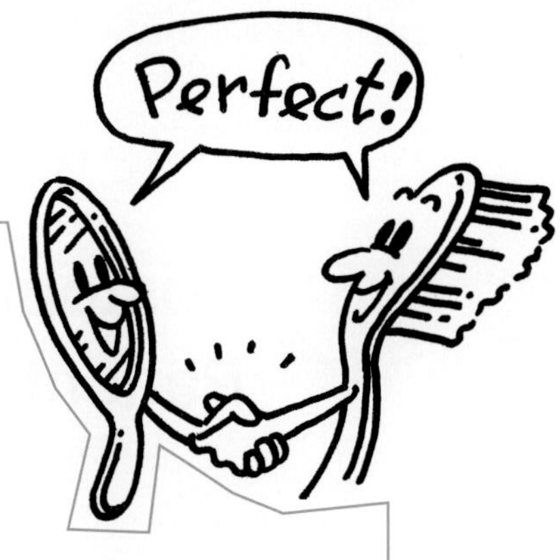

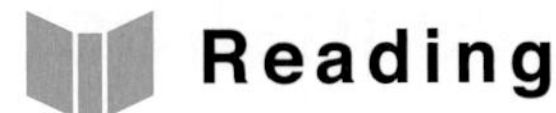

Reading

Proper brushing（適切なブラッシング方法）

The most efficient, simple and comfortable method to eliminate dental plaque at the individual's level is brushing A bad brushing technique might damage your teeth or gums. There are many different toothbrushing techniques available and it is best to ask your dental professionals to advise you of the one that is right for you. You should replace your toothbrush about every 2 to 3 months. Worn out or shaggy toothbrushes are not so effective in removing plaque from the teeth.

The following brushing instructions can be used as a guide.
Brush your teeth systematically: start with the outer surfaces, next the inner surfaces and lastly the chewing surfaces. Always start with the back teeth as they are most difficult to clean.

1. Tilt the bristles of the toothbrush along the gumline at an angle of 45 - or 90 -degree. Bristles should contact softly both the tooth surface and the gumline.
2. Gently brush the outer tooth surfaces of 2 - 3 teeth with short, vibratory back and forth strokes, so the tips of the bristles stay in one place. Do this for about 20 to 30 strokes. This assures that adequate time will be spent cleaning away as much plaque as possible. Move brush to the next group of 2 - 3 teeth and repeat. Pay particular attention to the gumline. Using the correct angle and brushing action, clean all outer surfaces of upper and lower teeth making sure the bristles get into the spaces between teeth.
3. For cleaning the inner surfaces of the back teeth, maintain a 45 -degree angle with bristles contacting the tooth surface and gumline. Gently brush using light back and forth motion along all of the inner tooth surfaces.
4. For cleaning the inner surfaces of the front teeth, where the horizontal brush position is cumbersome, tilt the brush vertically behind the front teeth. Make several up and down strokes using the tip (front half) of the brush.
5. To clean the biting or chewing surfaces of the teeth, place the brush against the biting surface of the teeth and use a short back and forth scrubbing motion.

Q1 How many times do you brush your teeth in a day?
Q2 Who will provide proper tooth brushing instruction?
Q3 How often do I have to change my toothbrush?

263-00488

15 Postoperative Instructions to the Patient

Part I

Warm up

After completion of treatment, it is often the responsibility of the dental assistant or dental hygienist to give postoperative instructions to the patient. Although it is easy to forget to do this, the instructions are often very much appreciated by the patient. If the patient is a child, the parent must also be present when the instructions are given.

Vocabulary

postoperative 〈形〉診察後の，手術後の
prophylaxis 〈名〉予防
composite resin 〈名〉コンポジットレジン，複合レジン
mandibular 〈形〉下顎の
numbness 〈名〉麻痺，無感覚，しびれ
　cf. numb 〈形〉麻痺した，無感覚の
wear off 〈動〉（麻酔などが）切れる，次第になくなる
gently 〈副〉やさしく，ゆるやかに
anesthetic 〈名〉麻酔薬
amalgam 〈名〉アマルガム
immediately 〈副〉すぐに，即座に
require 〈動〉必要とする，要求する
bite 〈動〉かむ
yogurt (yoghurt) 〈名〉ヨーグルト

263-00488

Dialogue

音声：15_Part1-D.mp3

Situation Mr. Khan has just received oral prophylaxis and a composite resin filling in a mandibular second molar. The dental hygienist, Ms. Matsubara, is giving postoperative instructions.

Ms. Matsubara（M） Dr. Yamahira has asked me to give you postoperative instructions.

Mr. Khan（K） When will the numbness wear off?

M It usually takes about two or three hours.

K Is there anything I can do to make it go away faster?

M You might try to gently massage the jaw, but don't worry, the anesthetic will wear off naturally.

K Do I have to wait one day before I can eat on the tooth?

M This was true for amalgam fillings, but composite resin is hard immediately after the light is placed on it.

K That's good.

M You can use it as soon as the anesthetic wears off.

K But I am hungry now.

M You should not eat anything that requires chewing because you might bite your lip or tongue and not know it.

K Can I drink juice or something?

M It is fine to drink or eat something like yogurt or soup that does not require chewing.

263-00488

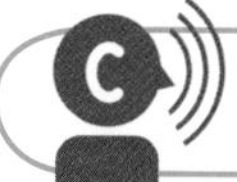

Listening 質問を聞いて，正しい答えを選びましょう

音声：15_Part1-L.mp3

1. *a* For half an hour.
   b For a few hours.
   c For half a day.

2. *a* As soon as the anesthetic wears off.
   b One hour after the anesthetic wears off.
   c Tomorrow.

3. *a* Because his tooth is not hard enough.
   b Because he might unconsciously bite his tongue or lip.
   c Because his jaw is weak now.

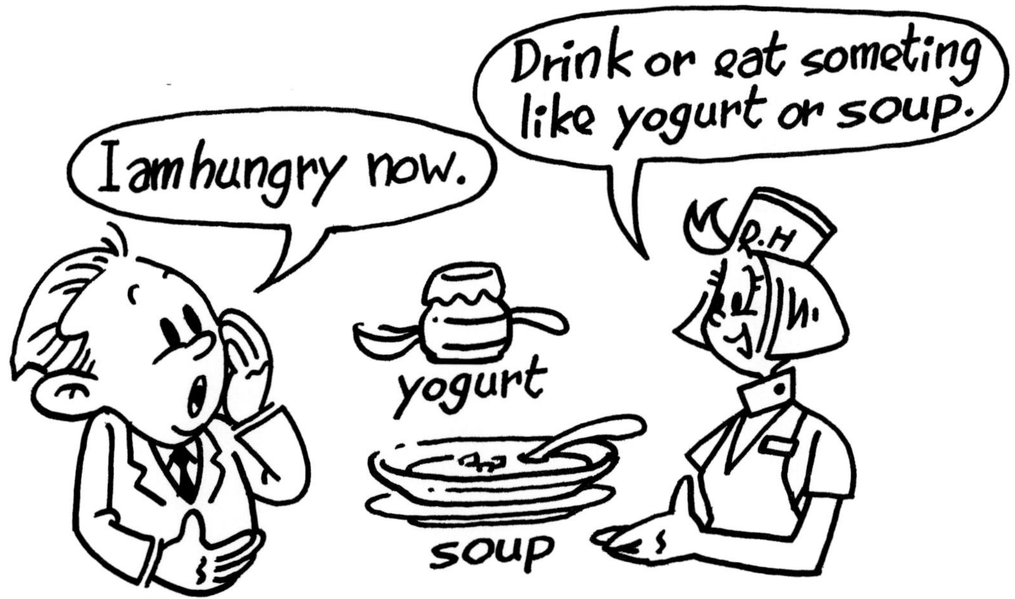

I am hungry now.
Drink or eat someting like yogurt or soup.
D.H
yogurt
soup

263-00488

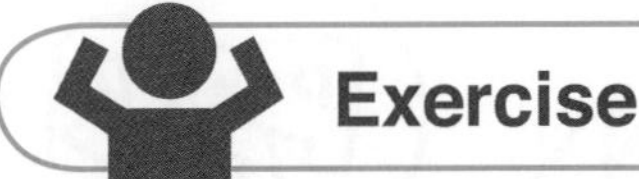

Exercise

Dialogue に出てきた表現を使って作文してみましょう.

① Is there anything I can do to ～ ?
（～するために私にできることはありますか？）

（例）

Is there anything I can do to make it go away faster?
（それ（＝麻酔）が早く切れるように何かできることはありますか？）
Is there anything I can do to help you finish the work sooner?
（少しでも早くあなたの仕事が終わるように私にできることはありますか？）

Is there anything I can do to ______________________________?

② You can ～ as soon as …
（…したらすぐに～することができます／してもよいです）

（例）

You can use it as soon as the anesthetic wears off.
（麻酔が切れたらすぐにそれ (= 歯) を使うことができます.）
You can start eating as soon as everybody gets back home.
（全員が帰ってきたらすぐに食べ始めていいですよ.）

You can ____________________ as soon as ____________________.

③ It is fine to ～ .（～するのはかまいません／～しても大丈夫です）

（例）

It is fine to drink or eat something like yogurt or soup.
（ヨーグルトやスープのようなものを食べたり飲んだりするのはかまいません.）
It is fine to make mistakes when you speak a foreign language.
（外国語を話すときにまちがえても大丈夫です.）

It is fine to ____.

263-00488

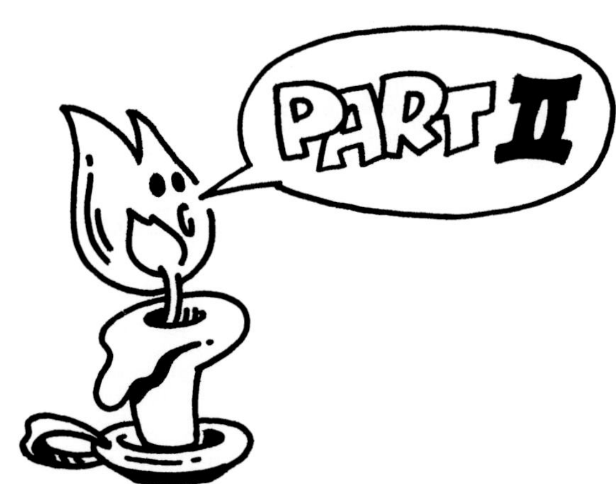

Part II

Warm up

This is a continuation of the previous dialogue.

Vocabulary

burn 〈動〉焼く，火傷を起こす
sore 〈形〉痛い，ひりひりする
sensitive 〈形〉敏感な，傷つきやすい　***cf.*** sensitivity 〈名〉敏感さ
region 〈名〉部位，領域
expose ～ to … 〈動〉～を…にさらす
fluids 〈名〉分泌液，流体
decrease 〈動〉減らす
desensitize 〈動〉感覚を鈍らせる

263-00488

 Dialogue

音声：15_Part2-D.mp3

Situation The dental hygienist, Ms. Matsubara, is giving postoperative instructions to Mr. Kahn.

Ms. Matsubara（M） You should be careful not to drink anything too hot before the numbness wears off.

Mr. Kahn（K） Why is that?

M Hot drinks like coffee could burn your lip and you would not know it if your lip is numb.

K What should I do if my gums are sore from the cleaning?

M Since you did not have a cleaning for two years, your gums and teeth may be a bit sensitive tomorrow.

K Yes. I expect that.

M Please brush with a soft bristled toothbrush and be gentle on the gums.

K Should I take Tylenol if I have pain?

M That would be fine, if you think you need it. Also, your teeth might be a bit sensitive to cold.

K Why is that?

M Calcium deposits have been removed from the region of the teeth near the gum line. This may cause sensitivity because it exposes the teeth to fluids in the mouth.

K How long will the sensitivity last?

M It will usually go away in a few days.

K Is there anything I can do to decrease the sensitivity?

M The best thing is to brush with desensitizing toothpaste.

K Thank you for telling me about this.

263-00488

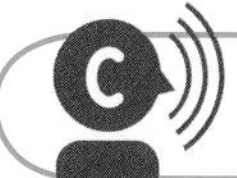

Listening 質問を聞いて，正しい答えを選びましょう

音声：15_Part2-L.mp3

1. *a* Cold drinks.
   b Hot drinks.
   c Sweet drinks.

2. *a* He can take it depending on his condition.
   b He should definitely take it after he gets home.
   c He must not take it even if he has pain.

3. *a* To brush with a soft bristled toothbrush.
   b To brush with desensitizing toothpaste.
   c To brush at least three times a day.

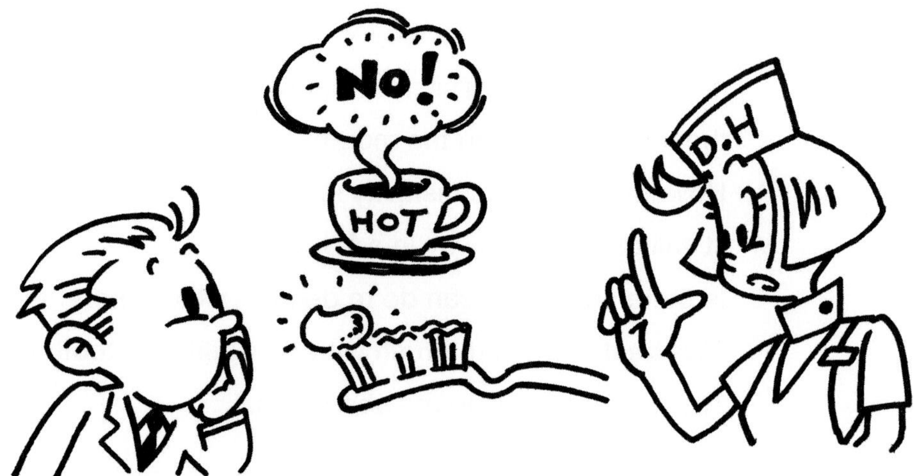

263-00488

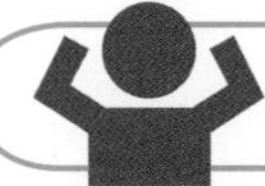

Exercise

① Dialogue に出てこなかった内容で，患者さんが診察後に歯科衛生士にたずねる可能性のある質問を英語で書いてみましょう（箇条書きで）.

・

・

・

・

・

② Dialogue に出てこなかった内容で，歯科衛生士が診察後の患者さんに行う指導として考えられる文章を英語で書いてみましょう（箇条書きで）.

・

・

・

・

・

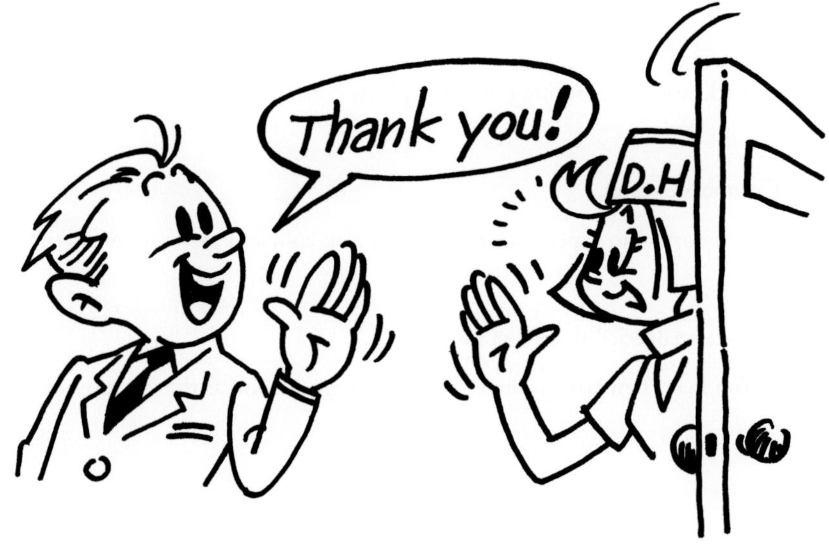

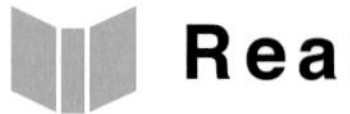

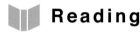

Reading

Post operative instructions（術後の注意）

When an anesthetic is used, your lips and tongue may be numb after the treatment. The length of time your mouth stays numb will depend on the type of anesthetic, and on how much the dentist gives you. Avoid any chewing and hot beverages until the numbness completely wears off. It is very easy to bite or burn your tongue, cheeks, or lips while you are numb. The numbness should go away within a few hours.

Endodontics:

・Your tooth and gum tissue may be slightly tender for several days. This tenderness is normal and is no cause for alarm.
・Do not chew food on the affected tooth until the treatment is completed.
・Discomfort may be alleviated by taking analgesics as directed. If you experience swelling, it may be necessary to take an antibiotic. Alcohol intake is not advised while taking these medications.
・If you experience discomfort that cannot be controlled with the above listed medications, or swelling develop, please contact the dentist immediately.

Composite resin:

・It is normal to experience some slight hot, cold and pressure sensitivity for a few days.
・Take analgesics as needed for pain.
・You may chew with your composite fillings as soon as the anesthetic completely

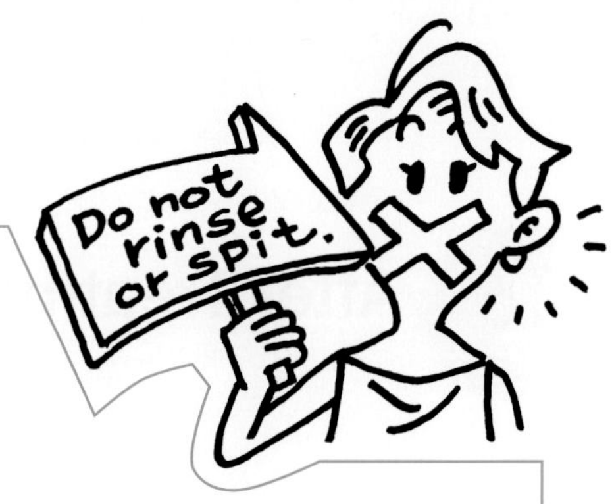

wears off, since they are fully set when you leave the operatory.

- If your bite feels uneven or if you have persistent pain, please call the dentist.

Tooth extraction:

- Do not rinse or spit for 24 hours after surgery.
- Apply an ice pack to the outside of your face in the surgical area for first 12 hours, apply ice 20 minutes on and 10 minutes off alternately.
- Some discomfort is normal after surgery. For pain or swelling take analgesics or antibiotics.
- Take soft foods which can be easily chewed and swallowed. Drink plenty of fluids, but do not use a straw.
- Do not smoke for at least 12 hours after surgery. Nicotine may break down the blood clot and interfere with healing.
- Some bleeding is expected after surgery. Bleeding is controlled by applying pressure to the extraction site using small rolled gauze. If bleeding still persists call the dentist.

Q1 What advice is necessary for patients after local anesthesia?

Q2 Is it common to experience slight pain after dental treatment?

Q2 What patients should do if symptoms persist?

263-00488

16 After Treatment

Warm up

After the patient has completed his appointment there are three important things that the receptionist must do. The patient should be given any medicine the dentist has prescribed, the next appointment should be scheduled, and the fee for the treatment should be collected.

Vocabulary

prescribe 〈動〉処方する
schedule 〈動〉予定をたてる
fee 〈名〉料金，費用
collect 〈動〉徴収する，集める
impression 〈名〉印象

263-00488

Dialogue

音声：16-D.mp3

Situation Ms. Wright has just completed an appointment where she had a tooth prepared for a crown and an impression taken. The receptionist, Ms. Kitamura, is talking with her.

Ms. Kitamura（K） How was your treatment today?

Ms. Wright（W） Actually, it wasn't as bad as I thought it would be.

K That's good. The doctor ① has asked me to give you this medicine.

W Thank you. What is it?

K It is Voltaren for pain. Take one or two tablets every five or six hours if you need it.

W Is it necessary to ② take it if I don't have a problem?

K No. Only take it if you think you need to.

W Dr. Kim ③ was very gentle, so I don't think I'll need to take the medicine. But thank you for giving it to me.

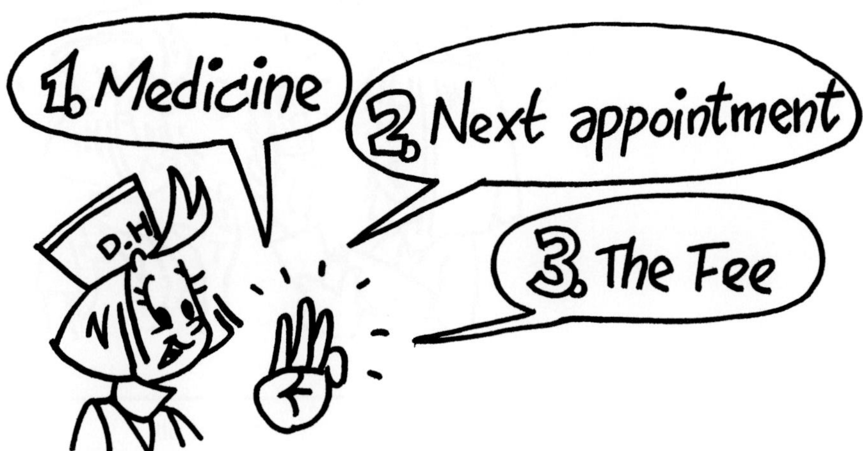

①	Dr. Lee	Dr. Brown
②	Do I still have to	Should I still
③	Dr. Lee	Dr. Brown

（Pair Work 参照）

263-00488

K You're welcome. ④ The next appointment will be in two weeks for putting in the crown. Would Thursday, April 7th, ⑤ be good for you?

W Yes, that is fine. Could I come in at 9:00 am? ⑥

K That time is taken. Would 10:00 am be acceptable?

W That would be fine. How long is the appointment?

K It will take about thirty minutes. ⑦

W I am looking forward to getting the new crown.

K I am sure you will be happy with it. The fee today is 20,000⑧ yen.

W Is it OK to pay by credit card?

K Certainly.

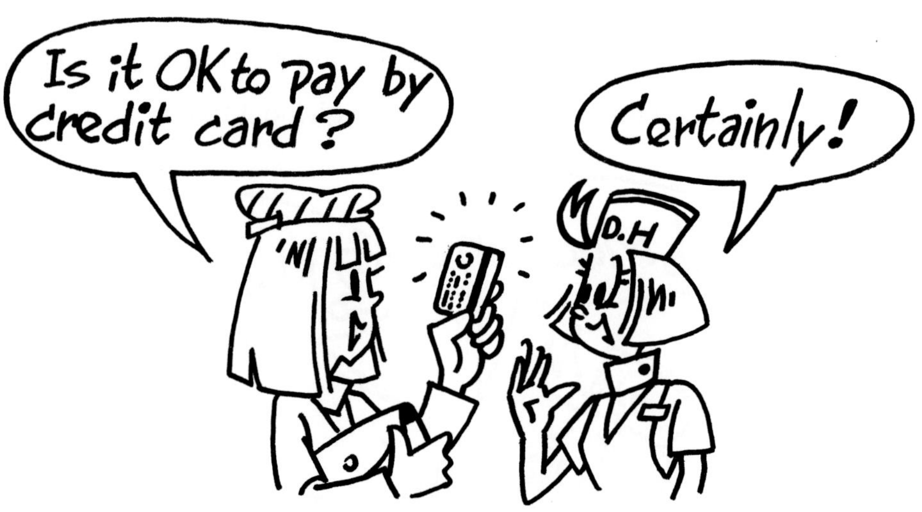

④	Sure	Not at all
⑤	Monday, January 22nd	Wednesday, October 30th
⑥	11:00am	noon
⑦	twenty minutes	half an hour
⑧	9,800	17,500

(Pair Work 参照)

263-00488

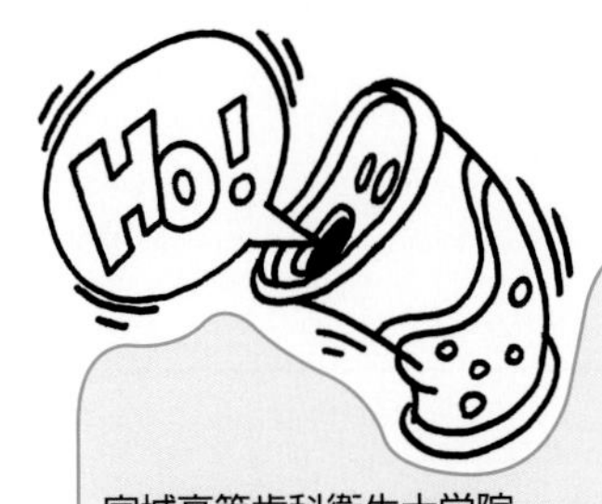

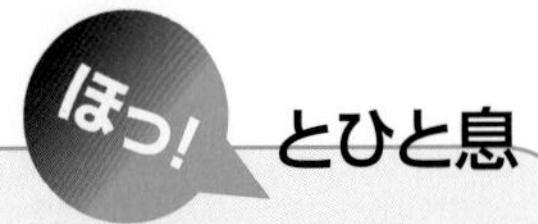

歯科衛生ケアプロセスと北米の歯科衛生士

宮城高等歯科衛生士学院
佐藤陽子

臨床で患者さんに接するときには，それまで勉強し，経験してきたことをもとに，指導者である歯科衛生士や歯科医師の対応を参考にしながら，その患者さんが最も必要とする関わりをしたいと願うものです．その際，学んできた知識を実際の臨床に効果的に活かすような考え方が必要になります．

歯科衛生ケアプロセス（dental hygiene process of care）とは，歯科衛生士の臨床・教育の骨格をなす概念であり，アセスメント（assessment），歯科衛生診断 (dental hygiene diagnosis)，計画立案（planning），実施（implementation），評価（evaluation）の5つの段階で構成されるものです．歯科衛生ケアプロセスは，対象となる人のことを考える思考の過程（process）であり，対象者のニーズに応じた科学的な根拠に基づいたケア（care）を行うことを目指しています．科学的な意思決定と問題解決が，歯科衛生ケアプロセスを支える2本柱となります．

北米の歯科衛生士は，この概念をもとに教育を受け，臨床に従事し，社会的なポジションを獲得してきました．具体的には，米国歯科衛生士会が，1993年に発表したポリシーマニュアル「理論構築の枠組み」のなかで歯科衛生の専門性を定義し，歯科衛生ケアプロセスに基づいた専門職の業務モデルを提示しました．以来，歯科衛生ケアプロセスは，臨床・教育の基盤となっています．また，カナダでは，歯科衛生士教育プログラムの認定条件のなかに，卒業時の学習成果として歯科衛生ケアプロセスが含まれています．歯科衛生ケアプロセスは，歯科衛生士の臨床の基本概念であり，カナダ歯科衛生士会により明確に定義されています．

現在，米国では，業務範囲を拡大した上級実践歯科衛生士（Advanced Dental Hygiene Practitioner: ADHP）制度が準備され，また，カナダでは，高齢者施設などにおいて歯科医師の監督なしに歯科衛生ケアを実施できるレジデンシャルケア歯科衛生士（Residential Care Dental Hygienist）制度が成功しています．いずれも歯科衛生士の意思決定・問題解決能力を重視しており，歯科衛生士の専門性がさらに向上することが期待されています．その根底には，歯科衛生ケアプロセスを基盤とした教育と実践の積み重ね，そして歯科衛生独自の視点を重視した歯科衛生理論，概念モデルの構築のための努力があるということを知っておいてほしいと思います．

263-00488

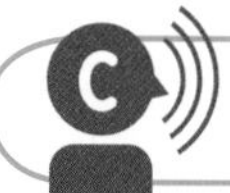

Listening 質問を聞いて，正しい答えを選びましょう

音声：16-L.mp3

1. *a* Not more than two.
   b At least three.
   c As many as she wants.

2. *a* April 7th, 9am.
   b April 7th, 10am.
   c April 17th, 10am.

3. *a* In cash.
   b By credit card.
   c By check.

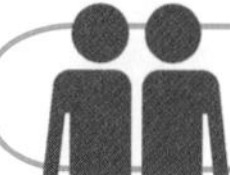

Pair Work

ペアになり，下線部を入れ替えて Dialogue を練習しましょう．

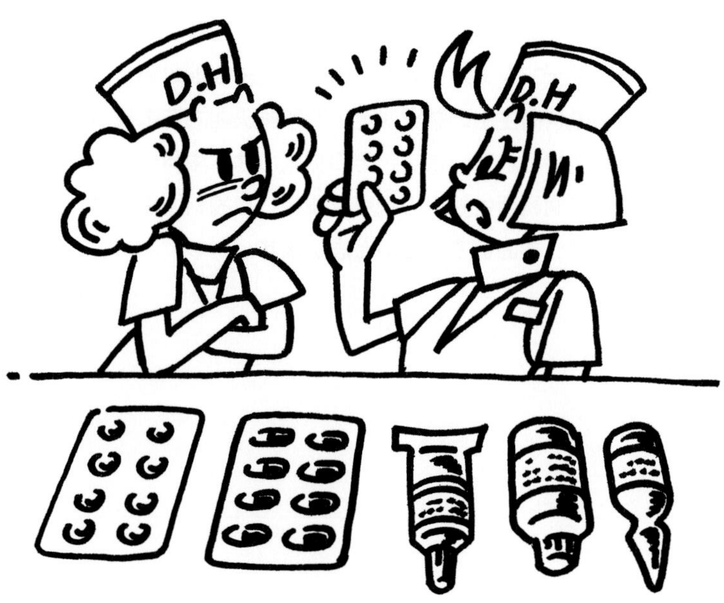

263-00488

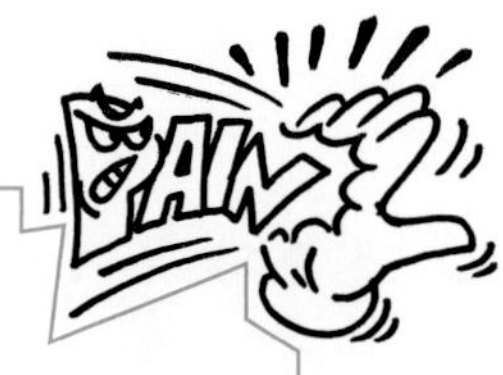

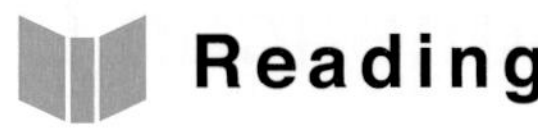

Reading

Common medication for dental pain（歯科でよく使われる鎮痛剤）

Non-narcotic analgesics or painkillers are the most commonly used drugs for relief of toothache or pain following dental treatment. This category includes aspirin, acetaminophen and ibuprofen.

Aspirin:
Aspirin remains one of the most popular drugs for treating mild to moderate pain. The primary function of aspirin is to reduce pain, swelling and fever.
It is unsure exactly how the substance works, but it is known that it prevents pain by acting on the hypothalamus and blocking the generation of pain impulses. It also reduces inflammation by inhibiting prostaglandin production.
One important side effect of aspirin is that it can increase bleeding. This is of critical importance to a dentist who is performing surgical procedures, such as tooth extractions, scaling and root plaining, gingival surgery, and biopsies. The daily use of aspirin can cause excessive and prolonged bleeding during and after these procedures. In some cases, aspirin should be avoided prior to dental procedures. The decision to alter aspirin intake should be made with the consultation of a doctor and a dentist. Some people find that taking aspirin upsets their stomach. To avoid this, patients should take aspirin with meals, or a full glass of water or milk.

Acetaminophen:
Acetaminophen is widely used over-the-counter drugs which reduce pain and fever. Dentists generally use it for mild to moderate dental pain and generally safe for acute dental pain. It acts as both anti-pain and anti-fever, but has little anti-inflammatory action.
It is believed that the drug may increase a patient's pain threshold by blocking pain centers in the central nervous system.
Though acetaminophen is often a safe and effective painkiller, it causes liver damages at very high single doses. It is generally gentler on the stomach than aspirin. However, in some patients, acetaminophen can cause upset stomach. To help avoid this problem, patients may be advised to take acetaminophen with meals or milk. It is important to note that caffeine increases the effect of acetaminophen.

Ibuprofen:
Ibuprofen relieves mild to moderate pain, inflammation, and swelling.
It is unknown exactly how ibuprofen works. However, it is believed that ibuprofen works by inhibiting the enzyme that makes prostaglandins, resulting in lower levels of prostaglandins.
Certain conditions may raise concerns for patients taking ibuprofen. Patients who have ulcers or who experience gastrointestinal upset when taking aspirin should not take ibuprofen. In general, ibuprofen is a safe drug that causes few side effects in most people. However, ibuprofen sometimes causes upset stomach, although it is usually gentler on the stomach than aspirin. To avoid upsetting the stomach, ibuprofen can be taken with food or milk.

263-00488

17 Visit to an American Dental Clinic

Part I

Warm up

Visiting dental offices in Japan and abroad can be very educational.

Vocabulary

educational 〈形〉教育上有益な
friendly 〈形〉親しげな，友好的な
group practice 〈名〉チーム医療
manage 〈動〉管理する，対処する
run 〈動〉運営する，取り仕切る
incorporated 〈形〉法人組織の，会社組織の
general practitioner 〈名〉一般歯科医
pedodontist 〈名〉小児歯科医
prosthodontist 〈名〉補綴歯科医
periodontist 〈名〉歯周病専門医
specialist 〈名〉専門医，専門家
decathlon 〈名〉（陸上の）十種競技
dentistry 〈名〉歯科医療，歯科学
refer 〈動〉照会させる，任せる

263-00488

Dialogue

音声：17_Part1-D.mp3

Situation Junko Takeuchi, a dental hygienist from Sapporo is visiting a dental office in San Francisco. She is talking with the office manager, Mary Boyd.

Junko (J) Thank you Ms. Boyd for inviting me to visit your clinic.

Mary (M) Hi, Junko. I am glad you could come here. You can call me Mary.

J Being from Japan, I am not used to calling people by their first names.

M At our clinic we call everyone by his or her first name, even the patients. It seems friendlier that way.

J This is a big office. How many people work here?

M We have a group practice. There are five dentists and a staff of 23.

J Wow. That is a lot for you to manage. It seems like you are running a company.

M It is a company. Many large dental offices like this one are incorporated.

J Why are there so many dentists in one office?

M Two of the dentists are general practitioners, one is a pedodontist, one is a prosthodontist and one is a periodontist.

J In Japan a dentist is expected to do everything. There are very few specialists.

M That sounds like decathlon dentistry. In the US dentists often refer difficult cases to specialists so that the patient can have the best treatment possible.

J That sounds like a good idea.

263-00488

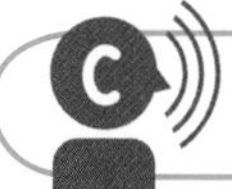

Listening 質問を聞いて，正しい答えを選びましょう

音声：17_Part1-L.mp3

1. *a* By her last name.
   b By her first name.
   c By her nickname.

2. *a* 5.
   b 23.
   c 28.

3. *a* Because Japanese dentists work longer hours than American dentists.
   b Because Japanese dentists have to do more things than American dentists.
   c Because Japanese dentists are physically stronger than American dentists.

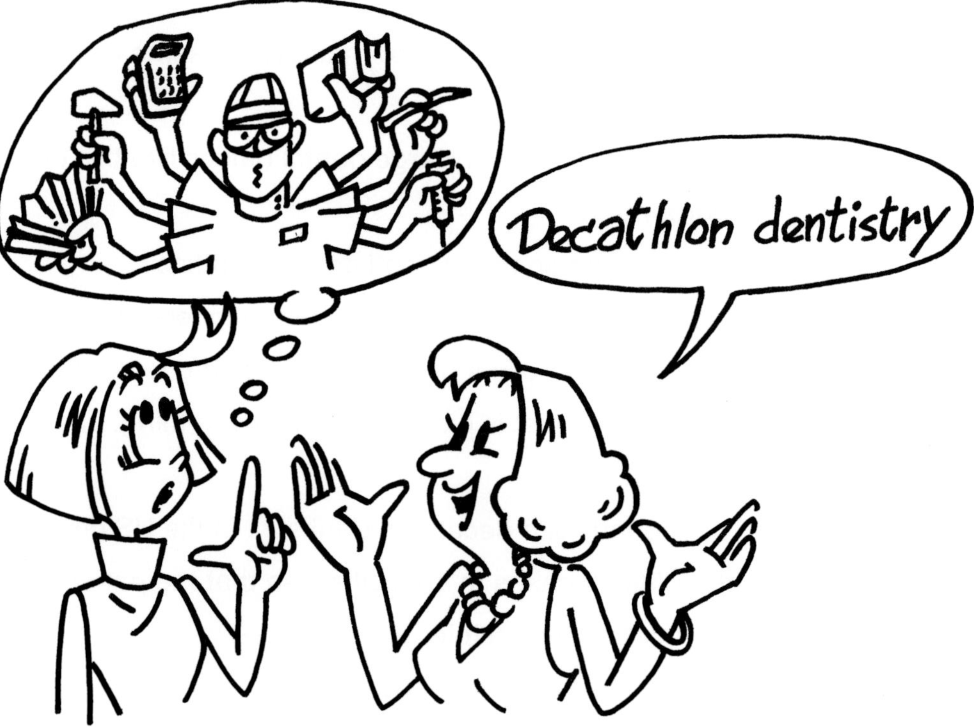

263-00488

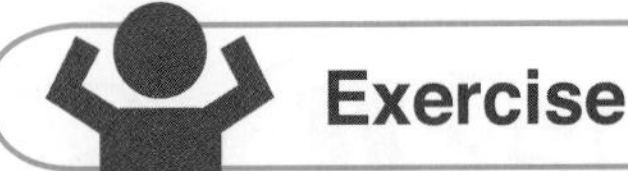

Exercise

Dialogue に出てきた表現を使って作文してみましょう.

① Thank you for ～ ing.（～してくれてありがとうございます）

（例）

Thank you for inviting me to visit your clinic.

（私をこちらのクリニックに招待してくださってありがとうございます.）

Thank you for coming to our presentation today.

（今日はわれわれの発表を聴きに来てくださりありがとうございます.）

Thank you for ______________________________.

② I am not used to ～ ing.（私は～することに慣れていません）

（例）

I am not used to calling people by their first names.

（ファーストネームで人をよぶことに慣れていません.）

I am not used to driving on the right side of the road.

（私は車で道の右側を走ることに慣れていません.）

I am not used to ______________________________.

263-00488

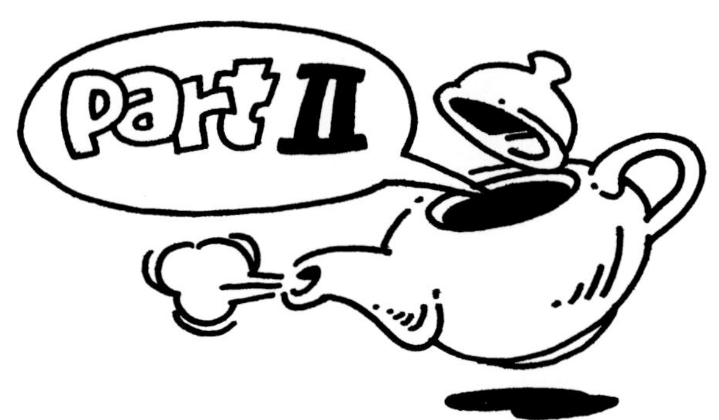

Part II

Warm up

This is a continuation of the previous dialogue.

Vocabulary

tour 〈名〉見学，旅行
sterilization 〈名〉消毒，滅菌，殺菌
private insurance 〈名〉(国民健康保険に対し) 民間保険会社による医療保険
root planing 〈名〉ルートプレーニング，根面清掃
certification 〈名〉免許
local anesthetic 〈名〉局部麻酔剤
responsibility 〈名〉責任
respected 〈形〉立派な，評判の高い
profession 〈名〉職業，専門職

263-00488

Dialogue

音声：17_Part2-D.mp3

Situation The office manager, Mary Boyd, is giving Junko Takeuchi a tour of the dental office.

Junko（J） Why do you need such a large staff here?

Mary（M） Three people work at the front desk, ten are dental hygienists, eight are dental assistants and two work full-time in sterilization.

J In the office where I work, I am expected to do everything.

M That sounds like decathlon dental hygiene!

J It is a lot of work. Do you accept national health insurance here?

M There is no national health insurance in the US. Most of the patients have private insurance.

J Could you show me one of the dental hygienist's rooms?

M Certainly. This is John's room.

J In Japan all dental hygienists are women.

M There are many male dental hygienists in the US now.

J Why does the dental hygienist have an assistant?

M Usually the dental hygienist works alone, but for difficult cases such as root planing, he has an assistant.

J If he is a dental hygienist, why is he giving anesthetic?

M Hygienists in California can receive training and certification to give local anesthetic.

J That is a lot of responsibility.

M Dental hygiene is a highly respected profession.

263-00488

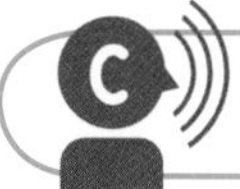

Listening 質問を聞いて，正しい答えを選びましょう

音声：17_Part2-L.mp3

1. *a* 3.
   b 8.
   c 10.

2. *a* National insurance.
   b Private insurance.
   c Both national and private insurance.

3. *a* To help the dental hygienist with difficult cases.
   b To help the receptionist at the front desk.
   c To give brushing instructions to the patient.

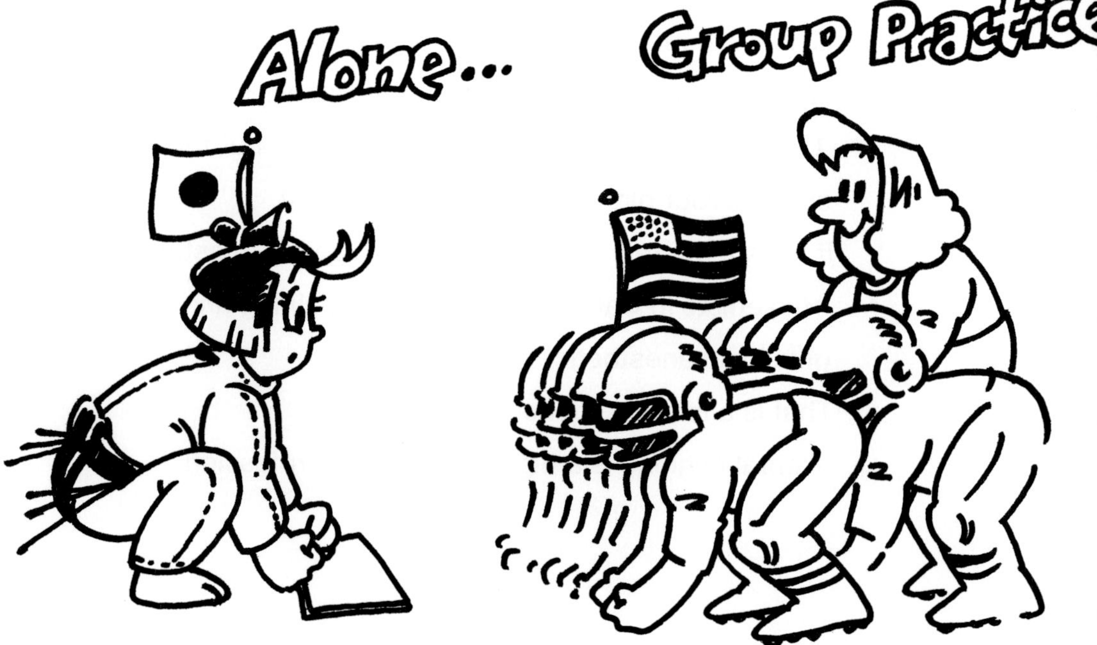

263-00488

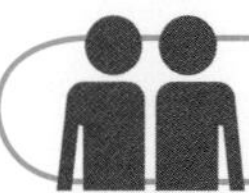

Pair Work

① Dialogue の内容，あるいは自分のもっている知識をもとに，日本と米国の歯科診療事情の違いについて英語で書いてみましょう．

日　本	米　国

② パートナーと答えを比べてみましょう．

263-00488

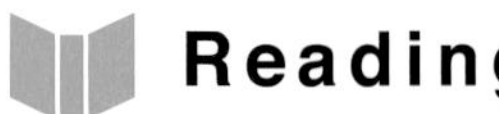

Reading

Dental hygienists in the world（世界の歯科衛生士）

In Japan, the law and regulation of dental hygienists was in active in 1948. In 1949, six schools started the training of dental hygienists and first dental hygienists graduated next year. After that the number of dental hygienists has been increasing and up till now more than 300,000 people got the license. In 2020, the number of practicing dental hygienist is about 143,000 in Japan. They are working at dental clinics, hospitals, health centers and education institutes.

The main three roles of Japanese dental hygienists are oral prophylaxis, health education and treatment assistance. Japan Dental Hygienists' Association is an official organization to represent and advance the profession of dental hygiene in Japan. It was established in 1951 and the number of members is 16,506 in 2020.

Not all the countries have the profession of dental hygiene and the roles of dental hygienists differ country by country. The International Federation of Dental Hygienists (IFDH) is an international organization, and it unites dental hygiene associations from around the world in their common cause of promoting dental health.

263-00488

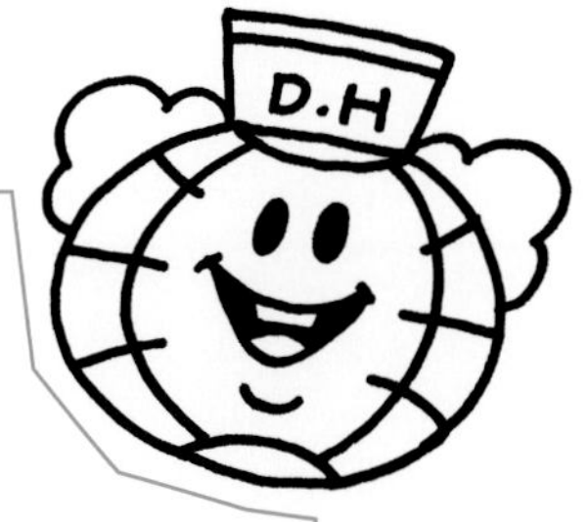

Association Members of the IFDH are the following.

Australia, Austria, Belgium, Canada, Cameroon, Czech Republic, Denmark Finland, Georgia, Germany, Ireland, Israel, Italy, Japan, Korea, Latvia Lithuania, Malta, Nepal, Netherlands, New Zealand, Norway, Portugal Russia, Singapore, Slovak Republic, South Africa, Spain, Sweden, Switzerland United Arab Emirates, United Kingdom, United States of America

Please visit the following web sites and check the oversea dental hygienist's activities.

IFDH	URL:http://www.ifdh.org/
The American Dental Hyienist' Association	URL:http://www.adha.org/
The British Dental Hygienists' Association	URL:http://www.bdha.org.uk/
The Canadian Dental Hygienists Association	URL:http://www.cdha.ca/
The Dental Hygienists Association of Australia	URL:http://dhaa.info/

Q1 What are the roles of dental hygienists in Japan?

Q2 How many dental hygienists are working now in Japan?

Q3 Are you a member of Japan Dental Hygienists' Association?

263-00488

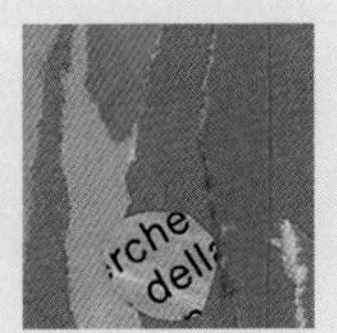

Part 2

Important Vocabulary for Dental Hygienists

1. 歯科医療に携わる者　Dental workforce

歯科医師	dentist
歯科衛生士	dental hygienist
歯科技工士	dental technician, dental technologist
歯科助手	dental assistant
歯科受付	dental receptionist

2. 歯科学　Dentistry

臨床歯科学	**Clinical dentistry**
予防歯科学	Preventive dentistry
口腔衛生学	Oral health
歯科保存学	Conservative dentistry
歯周病学	Periodontics, Periodontology
歯内療法学	Endodontics, Endodontology
歯科補綴学	Prosthodontics
口腔外科学	Oral surgery
歯科矯正学	Orthodontics
小児歯科学	Pedodontics, Pediatric dentistry
高齢者歯科学	Geriatric dentistry
歯科放射線学	Dental radiology
歯科麻酔学	Dental anesthesiology
社会歯科学	**Social dentistry**
地域歯科保健学	Community dentistry
歯科法医学	Dental forensic science
基礎歯科学	**Basic dentistry**
口腔解剖学	Oral anatomy
口腔生理学	Oral physiology

263-00488

口腔生化学	Oral biochemistry
口腔病理学	Oral pathology
口腔細菌学	Oral microbiology
歯科薬理学	Dental pharmacology
歯科理工学	Dental materials science and technology

3．検査　Examination

主訴	chief complaint
既往歴	anamnesis, medical history
現病歴	history of present illness
家族歴	family history
問診表	health questionnaire
問診	medical interview
視診	inspection
触診	palpation
打診	percussion
臨床検査	clinical examination
X線検査	roentgenographic (X-ray) examination
診断	diagnosis

4．痛みの種類　Pain

軽い痛み	slight pain
中等度の痛み	moderate (middle) pain
激しい痛み	severe (violent) pain
鋭い痛み	sharp pain
鈍い痛み	dull pain

急激な痛み	acute pain
拍動痛	throbbing (pulsating) pain
自発痛	spontaneous pain
持続痛	continuous pain
間歇痛	intermittent pain
冷水痛	cold water pain
咬合痛	biting (occlusal) pain
夜間痛	pain in bed, night pain
圧痛	oppressive pain
打診痛	percussion pain
術後痛	postoperative pain
関連痛	referred pain

5. 全身疾患　Systemic disease

高血圧	hypertension (high blood pressure)
低血圧	hypotension (low blood pressure)
糖尿病	diabetes
結核	tuberculosis
胃潰瘍	gastric ulcer
肝炎	hepatitis
腎炎	nephritis
肺炎	pneumonia
虫垂炎	appendicitis
喘息	asthma
リューマチ熱	rheumatic fever
関節炎	arthritis
癌	cancer
貧血	anemia

263-00488

血友病	hemophilia
白血病	leukemia
エイズ	AIDS (acquired immunodeficiency syndrome)

6. 歯科疾患　Dental disease

齲蝕	dental caries
歯髄炎	pulpitis
歯肉炎	gingivitis
歯周炎	periodontitis
智歯周囲炎	pericoronitis
口内炎	stomatitis
埋伏歯	impacted tooth
先天的欠如歯	congenital anodontia
咬耗症	attrition
摩耗症	abrasion
楔状欠損	wedge-shaped defect
口蓋裂	cleft palate
口唇裂	cleft lip
開口障害	trismus
歯ぎしり	bruxism, grinding
顎関節症	temporomandibular joint dysfunction (disorder)
口臭	halitosis
不正咬合	malocclusion

7. 歯科治療　Dental treatment

レジン充填	resin filling
アマルガム充填	amalgam filling

インレー	inlay
鋳造冠	cast crown
固定橋義歯	fixed bridge
部分床義歯	partial denture
全部床義歯	full denture
窩洞形成	cavity preparation
印象採得	impression taking
咬合採得	bite taking
修理	repairing
試適	trial application
研磨	polishing
装着	setting
セメント合着	cementation (cementing)
咬合調整	occlusal adjustment
抜髄	pulpectomy
根管治療	root canal treatment
根管充塡	root canal filling
麻酔	anesthesia
抜歯	tooth extraction
縫合	suture
刷掃指導	tooth brushing instruction (TBI)
歯石除去	scaling
滅菌	sterilization
消毒	disinfection

263-00488

8．歯の名称

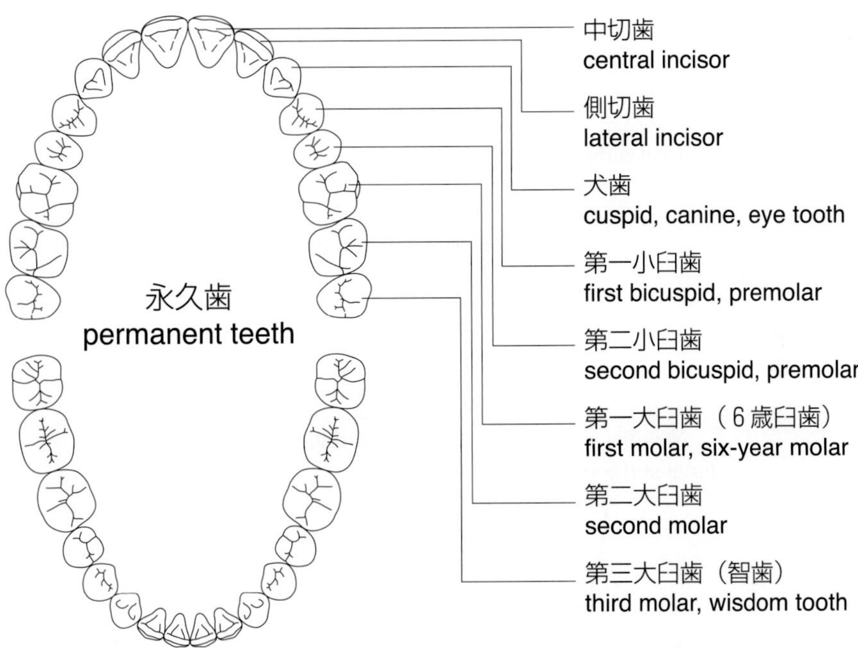

乳歯
deciduous teeth, milk teeth

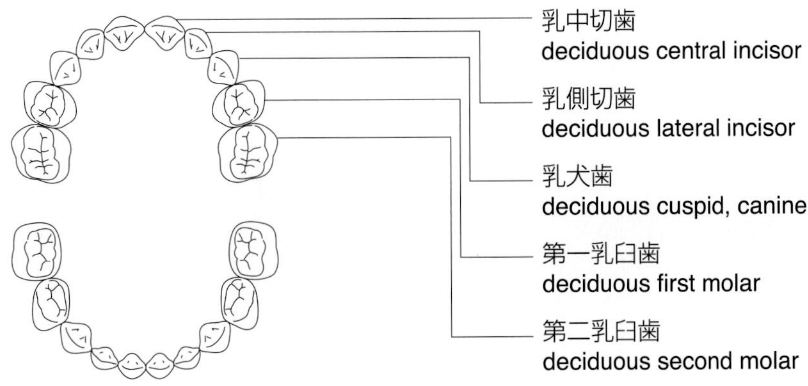

263-00488

9. 部位の名称　Word of direction

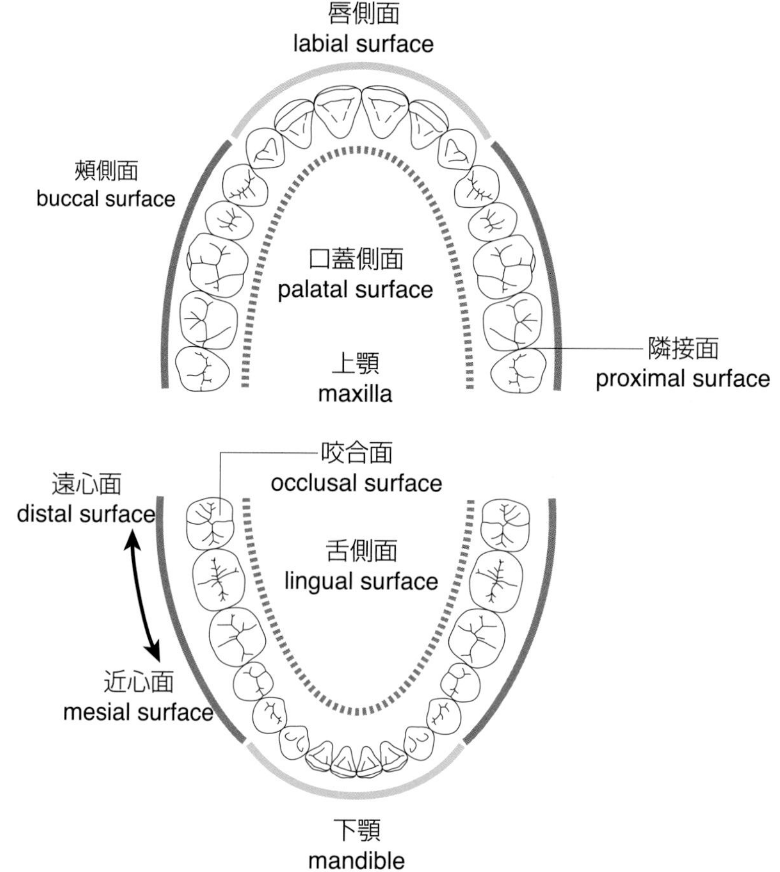

10. 口腔解剖用語　Dental anatomy

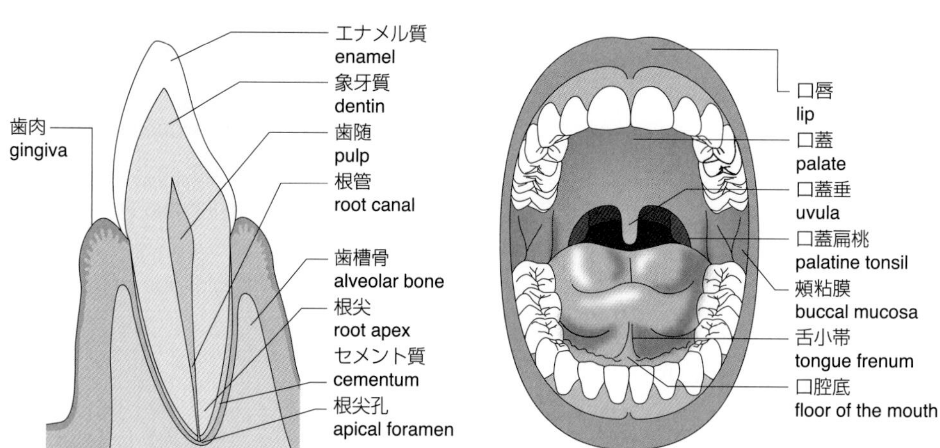

263-00488

11．人体各部位　Body

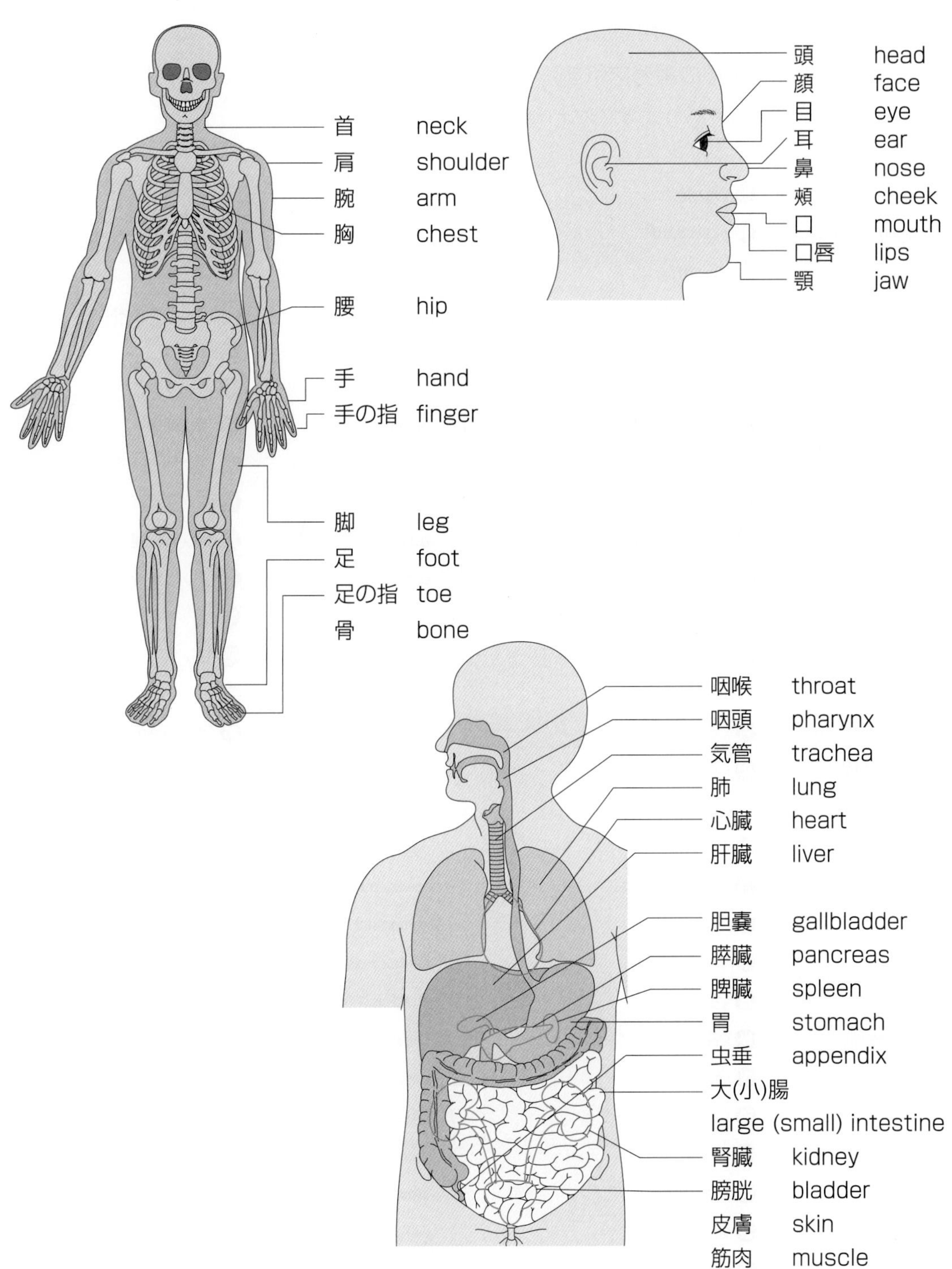
首 neck
肩 shoulder
腕 arm
胸 chest
腰 hip
手 hand
手の指 finger
脚 leg
足 foot
足の指 toe
骨 bone
頭 head
顔 face
目 eye
耳 ear
鼻 nose
頬 cheek
口 mouth
口唇 lips
顎 jaw
咽喉 throat
咽頭 pharynx
気管 trachea
肺 lung
心臓 heart
肝臓 liver
胆嚢 gallbladder
膵臓 pancreas
脾臓 spleen
胃 stomach
虫垂 appendix
大(小)腸
large (small) intestine
腎臓 kidney
膀胱 bladder
皮膚 skin
筋肉 muscle

263-00488

12. 歯科用頻出単語 296

ここに掲載する単語は，歯科関連の Web サイト（出典サイトについては巻末参照）から約 15 万語を抽出し，そのなかから使用頻度が多い 296 語を厳選したものです（アルファベット順．単語のあとの丸数字は頻出順の番号を示す）．使用法がわかりにくい単語（太字）については，リストの後に例文が掲載してあります．あわせて参照してください．

	単語	番号	意味
□	abrasion	279	〈名〉摩耗
□	abutment tooth	292	〈名〉支台歯
□	acid	79	〈名〉酸性
□	acute	237	〈形〉急性の
□	adjustment	238	〈名〉適応
□	**affect**	168	〈動〉影響を与える
□	**agent**	148	〈名〉作用物質
□	align	96	〈動〉調整する
□	allergic	250	〈形〉アレルギーの
□	allergy	71	〈名〉アレルギー
□	**alveolar**	216	〈形〉歯槽の
□	amalgam	117	〈名〉アマルガム
□	anesthesia	118	〈名〉麻酔
□	anesthetic	280	〈名〉麻酔薬
□	antibiotic	143	〈名〉抗生物質
□	**antimicrobial**	226	〈名〉抗菌薬
□	anxiety	210	〈名〉不安
□	**appliance**	204	〈名〉装置
□	appointment	176	〈名〉予約，約束
□	artificial	144	〈形〉人工的の
□	**asepsis**	165	〈名〉無菌状態
□	assessment	184	〈名〉評価
□	assurance	281	〈名〉保険
□	attached	251	〈形〉付着した
□	**attachment**	282	〈名〉アタッチメント
□	bacteria	26	〈名〉細菌
□	bacterial	252	〈形〉細菌性の
□	balanced	149	〈形〉平衡の
□	biofilm	283	〈名〉バイオフィルム
□	bite	211	〈名〉バイト
□	bite	268	〈動〉かむ
□	bleaching	82	〈名〉漂白法
□	bleed	260	〈動〉出血する
□	bleeding	77	〈名〉出血
□	bloodborne	97	〈形〉血液感染性の
□	bone	37	〈名〉骨
□	bracket	261	〈名〉ブラケット
□	breath	28	〈名〉呼吸
□	bridge	253	〈名〉架工義歯
□	bristle	177	〈名〉（ブラシなどの）毛
□	**bulimia**	254	〈名〉過食症
□	calcium	169	〈名〉カルシウム
□	calculus	101	〈名〉歯石
□	canal	98	〈名〉管
□	cancer	51	〈名〉癌
□	**cancerous**	40	〈形〉癌性の
□	**canker**	239	〈名〉潰瘍
□	caries	66	〈名〉カリエス，齲蝕
□	cavity	48	〈名〉窩洞，むし歯
□	**cavity margin**	72	〈名〉窩縁
□	cementum	212	〈名〉セメント質
□	central incisor	78	〈名〉中切歯
□	checkup	217	〈名〉検診
□	chew	178	〈動〉かむ
□	chewing	67	〈名〉咀嚼
□	**chief complaint**	52	〈名〉主訴
□	chronic	205	〈形〉慢性の
□	**clasp**	269	〈名〉鉤
□	cleaning	30	〈名〉クリーニング
□	clinic	218	〈名〉診療所
□	clinical	20	〈形〉臨床の
□	clinical trial	91	〈名〉臨床試験

263-00488

☐	**compliance**	227 〈名〉コンプライアンス
☐	composite resin	89 〈名〉コンポジットレジン
☐	connective tissue	85 〈名〉結合組織
☐	**consult**	186 〈動〉診察を受ける
☐	**contaminated**	179 〈形〉汚染された
☐	**contamination**	295 〈名〉汚染
☐	cosmetic dentistry	228 〈名〉審美歯科
☐	crown	109 〈名〉クラウン
☐	customary	187 〈形〉慣習上の
☐	damaged	284 〈形〉損傷した
☐	**debris**	219 〈名〉歯垢，残骸
☐	dental	1 〈形〉歯の
☐	dental hygienist	27 〈名〉歯科衛生士
☐	**dentifrice**	150 〈名〉歯磨剤
☐	dentin	151 〈名〉象牙質
☐	dentist	5 〈名〉歯科医師
☐	dentistry	25 〈名〉歯科
☐	denture	9 〈名〉義歯
☐	detect	240 〈動〉検出する
☐	**device**	107 〈名〉装置
☐	diabetes	75 〈名〉糖尿病
☐	diabetic	241 〈形〉糖尿病の
☐	diagnosis	58 〈名〉診察，診断
☐	diet	56 〈名〉食事
☐	**dietary**	145 〈形〉食事の
☐	discomfort	220 〈名〉不快，苦痛
☐	disease	7 〈名〉疾病
☐	**disinfectant**	293 〈名〉消毒剤
☐	disinfection	289 〈名〉消毒
☐	disorder	194 〈名〉疾患
☐	disposable	195 〈形〉ディスポーザブル
☐	drug	196 〈名〉医薬品
☐	**dry socket**	53 〈名〉ドライソケット
☐	effect	119 〈名〉効果
☐	effective	73 〈形〉効果的な
☐	enamel	42 〈名〉エナメル質
☐	**erosion**	296 〈名〉侵蝕症
☐	**evaluation**	54 〈名〉評価
☐	examination	120 〈名〉検査
☐	**exposure**	38 〈名〉被曝
☐	**extract**	152 〈動〉抜く
☐	extraction	270 〈名〉抜去
☐	factor	84 〈名〉因子
☐	filling	103 〈名〉充塡（物）
☐	film	157 〈名〉フィルム
☐	fissure	294 〈名〉裂溝
☐	fixed	153 〈形〉固定した
☐	floss	33 〈名〉フロス
☐	flossing	41 〈名〉フロッシング
☐	fluid	271 〈形〉流動性の
☐	**fluoridated**	129 〈形〉フッ素添加した
☐	fluoridation	114 〈名〉フッ化物添加
☐	fluoride	10 〈名〉フッ化物
☐	formation	255 〈名〉形成
☐	frequency	256 〈名〉頻度
☐	front teeth	154 〈名〉前歯
☐	gel	262 〈名〉ゲル
☐	gene	24 〈名〉遺伝子
☐	general anesthesia	68 〈名〉全身麻酔
☐	general practitioner	201 〈名〉一般医
☐	germ	242 〈名〉細菌
☐	gingival	121 〈形〉歯肉の
☐	**gingivitis**	81 〈名〉歯肉炎
☐	**grinding**	285 〈名〉研削
☐	guideline	59 〈名〉ガイドライン
☐	gum line	229 〈名〉歯肉ライン
☐	gums	15 〈名〉歯肉
☐	habit	197 〈名〉習癖
☐	halitosis	206 〈名〉口臭
☐	hand scaler	108 〈名〉手用スケーラー
☐	hard tissue	80 〈名〉硬組織
☐	healing	180 〈名〉治癒
☐	health	3 〈名〉健康
☐	health care	88 〈名〉医療
☐	healthy	43 〈形〉健康な
☐	hepatitis	76 〈名〉肝炎
☐	hygiene	17 〈名〉衛生
☐	illness	243 〈名〉疾患

	Word	No.	Meaning
☐	immediate	230	〈形〉即時の，緊急の
☐	impacted	221	〈形〉埋伏された
☐	implant	113	〈名〉インプラント
☐	impression	64	〈名〉印象
☐	incisor	83	〈名〉切歯
☐	index	23	〈名〉指数
☐	infected	286	〈形〉感染した
☐	infection	14	〈名〉感染
☐	**infectious**	130	〈形〉感染性の
☐	**inflammation**	263	〈名〉炎症
☐	initial	244	〈形〉初期の
☐	injury	188	〈名〉損傷
☐	instruction	172	〈名〉指導
☐	instrument	39	〈名〉器具
☐	**intake**	245	〈名〉摂取
☐	**interdental**	125	〈形〉歯間の
☐	**interproximal**	272	〈形〉隣接歯間の
☐	irritation	207	〈名〉刺激
☐	jaw	135	〈名〉顎
☐	**latex**	34	〈名〉ラテックス
☐	lesion	273	〈名〉損傷
☐	lip	173	〈名〉口唇
☐	local	55	〈形〉局所の
☐	**local anesthesia**	155	〈名〉局所麻酔
☐	lower	158	〈形〉下顎の
☐	maintenance	231	〈名〉メインテナンス
☐	**malocclusion**	287	〈名〉不正咬合
☐	management	208	〈名〉管理
☐	medical	46	〈形〉医学の
☐	medication	92	〈名〉薬物療法
☐	medicine	166	〈名〉薬剤
☐	metal	181	〈名〉金属
☐	missing	159	〈形〉欠落した
☐	molar	131	〈名〉大臼歯，臼歯
☐	monitoring	190	〈名〉モニタリング
☐	mouth	6	〈名〉口腔
☐	mouth rinse	274	〈名〉口内洗浄剤
☐	mouthguard	198	〈名〉マウスガード
☐	needle	275	〈名〉注射針
☐	normal	160	〈形〉正常な
☐	occupational diseases	182	〈名〉職業性疾患
☐	**odor**	126	〈名〉悪臭
☐	oral	4	〈形〉口腔の
☐	orthodontic	86	〈形〉歯列矯正の
☐	orthodontics	290	〈名〉歯科矯正学
☐	pain	62	〈名〉疼痛
☐	painful	222	〈形〉痛い
☐	palate	257	〈名〉口蓋
☐	partial denture	74	〈名〉部分床義歯
☐	particle	161	〈名〉粒子
☐	**pathogen**	104	〈名〉病原菌
☐	patient	18	〈名〉患者
☐	periodontal	16	〈形〉歯周の
☐	periodontitis	170	〈名〉歯根膜炎
☐	permanent	146	〈形〉永久の
☐	peroxide	276	〈名〉過酸化物
☐	personnel	191	〈名〉職員
☐	physician	112	〈名〉医師
☐	piercing pain	137	〈名〉ズキズキする痛み
☐	plaque	11	〈名〉歯垢
☐	plastic	183	〈名〉プラスチック
☐	polishing	232	〈名〉研磨
☐	post	156	〈名〉合釘
☐	practice	29	〈名〉診療
☐	**precaution**	132	〈名〉予防措置
☐	pregnancy	61	〈名〉妊娠
☐	pregnant	223	〈形〉妊娠している
☐	premolar	189	〈名〉小臼歯
☐	prescribe	246	〈動〉処方する
☐	prescription	224	〈名〉処方箋
☐	**prevent**	35	〈動〉予防する
☐	prevention	57	〈名〉予防
☐	preventive	115	〈形〉予防の
☐	primary	162	〈形〉原生の
☐	procedure	19	〈名〉手順，処置
☐	profession	213	〈名〉専門職
☐	professional	233	〈名〉専門家
☐	profile	36	〈名〉側貌

263-00488

□ **prophylaxis**	214	〈名〉予防
□ protection	199	〈名〉保護
□ protective dentin	185	〈名〉保護象牙質
□ protein	21	〈名〉タンパク質
□ pulp	49	〈名〉歯髄
□ questionnaire	234	〈名〉質問紙
□ radiation	147	〈名〉放射線
□ radiograph	105	〈名〉エックス線写真
□ rate	247	〈名〉比率
□ **recommendation**	94	〈名〉勧告
□ reduction	209	〈名〉還元
□ registered	248	〈形〉登録された
□ regularly	138	〈副〉規則的に，定期的に
□ **removable**	99	〈形〉可撤性の
□ **removal**	111	〈名〉除去
□ remove	277	〈動〉取り除く
□ **respiratory**	110	〈形〉呼吸の
□ **restoration**	65	〈名〉修復
□ **risk**	22	〈名〉リスク
□ root	31	〈名〉歯根
□ saliva	32	〈名〉唾液
□ salivary	225	〈形〉唾液の
□ scaling	123	〈名〉歯石除去
□ screening	264	〈名〉スクリーニング
□ sealant	90	〈名〉シーラント
□ **sedation**	235	〈名〉鎮静作用
□ sense	265	〈名〉感覚
□ sensitive	236	〈形〉敏感な
□ sensitivity	127	〈名〉感受性
□ signs	87	〈名〉徴候
□ smoking	174	〈名〉喫煙
□ solution	122	〈名〉溶液
□ sore	95	〈形〉痛い
□ stain	128	〈名〉ステイン，色素性沈着物
□ standard	163	〈形〉標準の
□ status	139	〈名〉状態
□ sterilization	215	〈名〉滅菌
□ sticky	200	〈形〉粘着性のある
□ stress	249	〈名〉応力，重圧

□ **substance**	13	〈名〉物質
□ supporting	164	〈形〉支持する
□ surface	50	〈名〉表面
□ surgery	93	〈名〉外科
□ surgical	192	〈形〉外科の
□ swelling	193	〈名〉腫脹
□ swollen	266	〈形〉腫れた
□ **symptom**	136	〈名〉症状，徴候
□ syndrome	267	〈名〉症候群
□ systemic	133	〈形〉全身性の
□ tartar	288	〈名〉歯石
□ taste	134	〈名〉味
□ **technique**	202	〈名〉方法
□ temporary	203	〈形〉一時的な
□ therapy	140	〈名〉療法
□ third molar	100	〈名〉第三大臼歯
□ tissue	47	〈名〉組織
□ tongue	44	〈名〉舌
□ tooth	2	〈名〉歯
□ tooth brushing	175	〈名〉ブラッシング法
□ tooth decay	12	〈名〉むし歯
□ toothbrush	45	〈名〉歯ブラシ
□ toothpaste	60	〈名〉歯磨剤
□ topical	116	〈形〉局所の
□ topical anesthesia	69	〈名〉表面麻酔
□ transmission	167	〈名〉伝染
□ treatment	8	〈名〉処置，治療
□ ultrasonic	141	〈形〉超音波の
□ upper	171	〈形〉上顎の
□ vaccination	258	〈名〉予防接種
□ vaccine	102	〈名〉ワクチン
□ vessel	278	〈名〉血管
□ virus	106	〈名〉ウイルス
□ waste	259	〈名〉廃棄物
□ whitening	124	〈名〉ホワイトニング剤
□ wisdom tooth	70	〈名〉智歯
□ **worn**	142	〈形〉摩耗した
□ **xerostomia**	291	〈名〉口腔乾燥症
□ X-ray	63	〈名〉エックス線写真

〈Example Sentences〉

affect: How does tobacco affect oral health?

agent: Bleaching agents are often applied to the teeth.

alveolar: The alveolar bone forms a socket around the tooth.

antimicrobial: Rinsing with antimicrobial mouth rinses may help reduce irritation.

appliance: Orthodontic appliances move teeth.

asepsis: Asepsis is essential during surgery.

attachment: The periodontal ligament forms an attachment between the teeth and bone.

bulimia: Bulimia is an eating disorder that is particularly destructive to teeth.

cancerous: Each year, cancerous growths of the mouth (oral cancer) develop in 30,000 people in the United States.

canker: Canker sores occur inside the mouth, and cold sores usually occur outside the mouth.

cavity margin: The cavity margin is where the filling meets the surface of the tooth.

chief complaint: The chief complaint is the main reason a patient seeks dental care.

clasp: Conventional partial dentures often have visible clasps.

compliance: Fluoride supplements require long-term compliance on a daily basis.

consult: If any problem persists, be sure to consult your dentist.

contaminated: Surgical instruments are often contaminated with blood.

contamination: Contamination of the wound should be avoided during surgery.

debris: Brush twice a day with a fluoride toothpaste to remove food debris and plaque.

dentifrice: There is no statistically significant difference between brushing with or without dentifrice.

device: A removable prosthetic device may be supported by implants.

dietary: Dietary sugars attack tooth enamel.

disinfectant: The dental chair is wiped with disinfectant.

dry socket: A dry socket may occur following extraction of a wisdom tooth.

erosion: Acidic foods may cause chemical erosion of the teeth.

evaluation: Every child should receive an orthodontic evaluation by age seven.

exposure: All workers must follow precautions to prevent occupational exposure to radiation.

263-00488

extract: It is often very difficult to extract third molars.

fluoridated: Fluoridated water is effective at reducing tooth decay.

gingivitis: Gingivitis is an infection within the gums caused by bacteria found in plaque.

grinding: Grinding the teeth at night may cause destruction of the enamel.

infectious: HIV is an infectious disease.

inflammation: Gingivitis is inflammation of the gums.

intake: Adequate fluid intake is important during hot weather.

interdental: An interdental brush is used to remove plaque from between the teeth.

interproximal: Plaque is difficult to remove in the interproximal areas.

latex: Surgical gloves are often made of latex.

local anesthesia: Dental hygienists are not allowed to administer local anesthesia.

malocclusion: Some examples of malocclusion are crowded teeth, extra teeth, missing teeth or jaws that are out of alignment.

odor: Brushing and flossing removes bacteria and reduces mouth odor.

pathogen: The dental staff should take care to prevent the spread of bloodborne pathogens.

precaution: As a precaution, dentists should receive hepatitis B vaccine.

prevent: Brushing helps prevent tooth decay.

prophylaxis: Oral prophylaxis is necessary to remove plaque and calculus.

recommendation: The dental hygienist gave her patients recommendations for toothbrushes.

removable: If you wear removable dentures, take them out at night.

removal: Bones and gums can shrink after the removal of teeth.

respiratory: Do you have any respiratory problems like a cough or difficulty breathing?

restoration: If the seal between the tooth enamel and the restoration breaks down, decay-causing bacteria may get under the restoration.

risk: Stress increases your risk of contracting an infection.

sedation: The patient is relaxed during conscious sedation.

substance: Plaque is a soft sticky substance that accumulates on teeth.

symptom: Bleeding around the teeth is a symptom of gum disease.

technique: Your dental hygienist can teach you proper brushing technique.

worn: It is important to replace worn dentures before they cause problems.

xerostomia: Halitosis is often caused by dry mouth (xerostomia), which occurs when the flow of saliva decreases.

13．患者さん向けの単語 52

専門用語	患者さん向け	日本語
abscess	infection in a tooth	膿瘍

An abscess can damage the bone around a tooth.
An infection in a tooth can damage the bone.

analgesic	pain medicine/pain killers	鎮痛薬

Analgesics do not increase the risk of hypertension.
Pain killers do not increase the risk of high blood pressure.

anterior tooth	front tooth	前歯

Dental implants make it possible to replace a single missing anterior tooth.
Dental implants make it possible to replace a single missing front tooth.

buccal	cheek side of the tooth	頬側の

The tooth surface directed toward the cheek is known as the buccal surface.
The tooth surface directed toward the cheek is known as the cheek side of the tooth.

calculus	calcium deposits on teeth	歯石

Dental calculus is a hard, stone-like material.
Calcium deposits on teeth are hard, stone-like material.

carcinoma	cancer	癌

Carcinoma can arise in the breast, colon, liver, lung, prostate, and stomach.
Cancer can arise in the breast, colon, liver, lung, prostate, and stomach.

cariogenic	decay producing	齲蝕原性の

Cariogenic bacteria produce acids.
Decay producing bacteria produce acids.

carious lesion	cavity/tooth decay	齲蝕病巣

Carious lesions destroy the tooth surface.
Tooth decay destroys (Cavities destroy) the tooth surface.

composite resin restoration	tooth-colored filling	コンポジットレジン修復

A composite resin restoration is an alternative to a traditional metal dental filling.
A tooth-colored filling is an alternative to a traditional metal dental filling.

crown	cap	クラウン

A gold crown covers the tooth.
A gold cap covers the tooth.

curette	instrument for cleaning teeth	キュレット

A curette is used to remove calculus from the root.
An instrument for cleaning teeth is used to remove calcium deposits from the root.

cusp	tip of the tooth	咬頭

Cusps are used to tear food.
The tips of teeth are used to tear food.

dental caries	cavity/tooth decay	齲蝕

Fluoride is effective in preventing dental caries.
Fluoride is effective in preventing cavities (tooth decay).

263-00488

歯科で使われる専門用語も，患者さんに使用する場合にはわかりやすい一般的な用語に置き換える必要があります．ここでは 52 の英単語を厳選しました．

専門用語	患者さん向け	日本語
dentifrice	toothpaste	歯磨剤

All patients are instructed to brush their teeth daily using a dentifrice and a toothbrush.
All patients are instructed to brush their teeth daily using toothpaste and a toothbrush.

dentition	teeth	歯列

The patient has an erupted permanent dentition.
The patient has erupted permanent teeth.

endodontic therapy	root canal treatment	根管処置

Endodontic therapy makes it possible to save teeth.
Root canal treatment makes it possible to save teeth.

first molar	six-year molar	第一大臼歯

A mandibular first molar requires endodontic therapy.
A lower six-year molar requires root canal treatment.

fixed prosthesis	bridge	架工義歯

A fixed prosthesis is used to replace missing teeth.
A bridge is used to replace missing teeth.

gingivitis	early gum disease	歯肉炎

Inflammation of the gingiva is called gingivitis.
Inflammation of the gums is called early gum disease.

halitosis	bad breath	口臭

Bacteria is the primary cause of halitosis.
Bacteria is the primary cause of bad breath.

impression	mold of the teeth	印象

A dental impression is a copy of the mouth made using an elastic material.
A mold of the teeth is a copy of the mouth made using an elastic material.

incisor	front tooth	切歯

Humans normally have eight incisors.
Humans normally have eight front teeth.

injection	shot	注射

The doctor will give you an injection to relieve the pain.
The doctor will give you a shot to relieve the pain.

lingual	tongue side of the tooth	舌側の

The lingual surfaces of the teeth easily collect plaque.
The tongue side of the teeth easily collect plaque.

malocclusion	misalignment of the teeth	咬合異常

Malocclusion is an orthodontic problem.
Misalignment of the teeth is an orthodontic problem.

mandible	lower jaw	下顎骨

The mandible consists of four major regions.
The lower jaw consists of four major regions.

専門用語	患者さん向け	日本語
maxilla	upper jaw	上顎骨

The maxilla forms the cheeks, nose, and roof of the mouth.
The upper jaw forms the cheeks, nose, and roof of the mouth.

molar	back tooth	大臼歯

Molars are used for grinding food.
Back teeth are used for grinding food.

occlusal surface	chewing surface	咬合面

The first molars have the largest occlusal surfaces of any of the teeth.
The six-year molars have the largest chewing surfaces of any of the teeth.

oral cavity	mouth	口腔

The two major afflictions of the oral cavity are dental caries and periodontal disease.
The two major diseases of the mouth are cavities and gum disease.

oral prophylaxis	teeth cleaning	歯口清掃

Oral prophylaxis removes plaque and calculus.
Teeth cleaning removes plaque and calcium deposits.

orthodontic treatment	braces	矯正治療

More adults are choosing to have orthodontic treatment to improve their appearance.
More adults are choosing to have braces to improve their appearance.

pedodontist	children's dentist	小児歯科医

A pedodontist is a dental specialist who treats only children.
A children's dentist is a dental specialist who treats only children.

periodontal disease	gum disease	歯周病

Periodontal disease is a major cause of tooth loss in adults.
Gum disease is a major cause of tooth loss in adults.

periodontal surgery	gum surgery	歯周外科

Periodontal surgery is recommended to correct or improve a periodontal problem.
Gum surgery is recommended to correct or improve a gum problem.

periodontal tissue	gums	歯周組織

Periodontal tissues surround the teeth.
The gums surround the teeth.

periodontist	gum disease specialist	歯周治療専門医

You should see a periodontist if you have periodontal disease.
You should see a gum disease specialist if you have gum disease.

pits and fissures	grooves in teeth	小窩裂溝

The dentist paints sealants over the pits and fissures on the surface of the teeth.
The dentist paints sealants over the grooves on the surface of the teeth.

pit and fissure sealant	sealant	小窩裂溝填塞材

You need pit and fissure sealants to help protect your teeth from decay.
You need sealants to help protect your teeth from decay.

263-00488

専門用語	患者さん向け	日本語
plaque	bacteria on teeth	歯垢

Periodontal disease is caused by plaque.
Gum disease is caused by bacteria on teeth.

posterior tooth	back tooth	後歯

The posterior teeth require strong fillings.
The back teeth require strong fillings.

primary dentition	baby teeth	乳歯列

The primary dentition consists of 20 teeth.
There are 20 baby teeth.

radiograph	X-ray	エックス線写真

A radiograph is an extremely important diagnostic tool.
An X-ray is an extremely important diagnostic tool.

removable prosthesis	removable denture	可撤性補綴装置

A removable prosthesis is cheaper than dental implants.
A removable denture is cheaper than dental implants.

restoration	filling	修復

Large restorations may cause sensitivity in the teeth.
Large fillings may cause sensitivity in the teeth.

root planing	deep cleaning	ルートプレーニング

Root planing is often necessary for periodontal disease.
Deep cleaning is often necessary for gum disease.

scaler	instrument for cleaning teeth	スケーラー

Calculus on the root surface is removed using a scaler
Calcium deposits on the root surface are removed using an instrument for cleaning teeth.

scaling	removal of calculus and deposits	歯石除去

Dental scaling should be done every six months.
Removal of calculus and deposits on the teeth should be done every six months.

subgingival	below the gum line	歯肉縁下の

Subgingival plaque causes periodontal disease.
Bacteria below the gum line cause gum disease.

supernumerary tooth	extra tooth	過剰歯

Sometimes a supernumerary tooth must be removed to facilitate the treatment of the remaining dentition.
Sometimes an extra tooth must be removed to facilitate the treatment of the remaining dentition.

temporomandibular joint	jaw joint	顎関節

The temporomandibular joint is the most complicated in the body.
The jaw joint is the most complicated in the body.

third molar	wisdom tooth	第三大臼歯

Third molars usually erupt in the late teens or early twenties.
Wisdom teeth usually erupt in the late teens or early twenties.

263-00488

14. 子ども向けの単語 19

専門用語	子ども向け	日本語
air turbine handpiece	tooth polisher	エアタービンハンドピース

The air turbine handpiece removes diseased tooth structure.
I will use the tooth polisher to clean your tooth.

専門用語	子ども向け	日本語
bacteria on teeth	germs on teeth/sugar bugs	歯の細菌

Bacteria cause tooth decay.
Germs on teeth (Sugar bugs) cause holes in the teeth.

専門用語	子ども向け	日本語
cavity/tooth decay	hole in the tooth	窩洞（むし歯）

The molar has a cavity.
Your back tooth has a hole in it.

専門用語	子ども向け	日本語
dental assistant	dental nurse	歯科助手

The dental assistant will help me clean your teeth.
The dental nurse will help me clean your teeth.

専門用語	子ども向け	日本語
dental hygienist	dental nurse	歯科衛生士

The dental hygienist will teach you how to brush.
The dental nurse will show you how to brush.

専門用語	子ども向け	日本語
examine teeth	count teeth	歯科検診をする

I would like to examine your teeth.
Shall we count your teeth?

専門用語	子ども向け	日本語
extract a tooth	wiggle out a tooth	抜歯する

The dentist will extract the tooth.
The dentist will wiggle out the tooth.

専門用語	子ども向け	日本語
floss	string	フロス

Floss can be used to clean between your teeth.
String can be used to clean between your teeth.

専門用語	子ども向け	日本語
injection/shot	medicine to make the tooth sleep	注射

I will give you an injection of anesthetic.
I will put medicine on your tooth to make it go to sleep.

専門用語	子ども向け	日本語
pain	discomfort	痛み

Let me know if you have any pain.
Let me know if you have any discomfort.

専門用語	子ども向け	日本語
pain medicine/pain killers	pills	錠剤

The dentist will give you pain medicine.
The dentist will give you pills.

専門用語	子ども向け	日本語
place sealant	put white plastic on teeth	シーラント

I will place sealants on the molars.
I will put white plastic on the back teeth.

専門用語	子ども向け	日本語
root canal treatment	clean inside the tooth	根管処置

I will do root canal treatment.
I will clean inside the tooth.

263-00488

前項に挙げた患者さん向けの単語を使用しても，子どもには通じないことが多いため，子どもにもわかりやすい単語に置き換える必要があります．ここでは 19 の単語を厳選しました．

専門用語	子ども向け	日本語
rubber dam	rubber raincoat	ラバーダム

The rubber dam will keep your mouth clean while I am working.
I will put a rubber raincoat on your tooth to keep your mouth clean.

専門用語	子ども向け	日本語
slow speed handpiece	tooth tickler	低速ハンドピース

The slow speed handpiece is used to remove tooth decay.
The tooth tickler polishes your tooth.

専門用語	子ども向け	日本語
stainless steel crown	silver tooth	乳歯用冠

I will put a stainless steel crown on the tooth to restore it.
I will make a silver tooth for you.

専門用語	子ども向け	日本語
tooth-colored filling	white plastic	歯の色をした充填物

Would you like a tooth-colored filling?
Would you like white plastic on your tooth?

専門用語	子ども向け	日本語
X-ray	picture of teeth	X線

I will take an X-ray of the teeth.
Let's take a picture of your teeth.

専門用語	子ども向け	日本語
X-ray machine	camera	X線装置

The X-ray machine exposes radiographs.
The camera takes pictures of your teeth.

263-00488

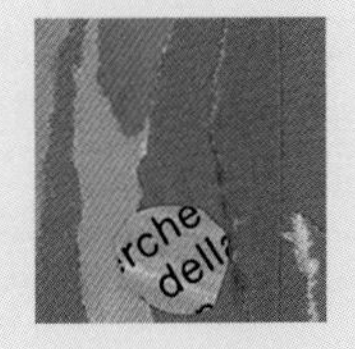

Part 3

歯科衛生士の仕事とは

歯科衛生士の仕事として，日本では「歯科衛生士法」第 2 条によって，①歯科疾患の予防処置，②歯科診療の補助，③歯科保健指導の 3 つが規定されています．では，外国では，歯科衛生士はどのような仕事をしているのでしょうか？　日本だけでなく，海外の同じ職業につく人たちに目を向けることは興味深いことです．そこで，ここでは英語圏の国，米国，英国，カナダの 3 カ国について調べてみます．

●米国の場合

まず取り上げるのは米国です．米国歯科医師会 (American Dental Association, ADA) のホームページ（http://www.ada.org/）をのぞいてみましょう．このホームページには「歯科衛生士カタログ (Dental Hygienist Brochure)」というセクションがあり，歯科衛生士のことを次のように説明しています（一部改変）．**Notes** を参考にして読んでみましょう．

Introduction

ここでは，歯科衛生士に関して基本的な事項，年齢・性別・人種に関係なく職業に就けること，最低 2 年間大学で教育を受けること，などが書かれています．

If you like helping people, enjoy working with your hands as well as your mind, and are interested in helping to prevent disease while assisting patients to maintain their health, a career as a dental hygienist may be for you.

Dental hygienists are important members of the dental health care team who work with dentists in the delivery of dental care to patients. Dental hygienists use their knowledge and clinical skills to provide dental hygiene care for patients. They use their interpersonal skills to motivate and instruct patients on methods to prevent oral disease and to maintain oral health.

Dental hygiene offers women and men of all ages, races and ethnic backgrounds exceptional career opportunities. A minimum of two years of college education

263-00488

that combines classroom and clinical coursework is necessary to become a dental hygienist. This education prepares graduates to provide care to patients in dental offices, clinics and educational or health care institutions. Studying in an accredited program provides education that is based on the latest procedures and techniques.

Dental hygienists are a valuable asset in a dental practice. In addition to performing technical duties, they play an important role in teaching patients appropriate oral hygiene techniques and counseling them regarding good nutrition and its impact on oral health.

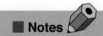

interpersonal skills 対人能力　**oral disease** 口腔疾患
ethnic backgrounds 民族的背景　**clinical** 臨床の
accredited program 認定プログラム　**valuable asset** 貴重な人材

What Do Dental Hygienists Do?

ここでは，歯科衛生士の職務内容を明確にしています．

A career as a dental hygienist offers a wide range of challenges.

In the dental office, the dentist and the dental hygienist work together to meet the oral health needs of patients. Since each state has its own specific regulations regarding their responsibilities, the range of services performed by dental hygienists varies from state to state. Some of the services provided by dental hygienists may include：

*patient screening procedures; such as assessment of oral health conditions, review of the health history, oral cancer screening, head and neck inspection, dental charting and taking blood pressure and pulse;

*taking and developing dental radiographs (X-rays);

*removing calculus and plaque (hard and soft deposits) from all surfaces of the teeth;

*applying preventive materials to the teeth (e.g., sealants and fluorides);

*teaching patients appropriate oral hygiene strategies to maintain oral health; (e.g., tooth brushing, flossing and nutritional counseling);

*counseling patients regarding good nutrition and its impact on oral health;

*making impressions of patients' teeth for study casts (models of teeth used by dentists to evaluate patient treatment needs); and

*performing documentation and office management activities.

Each state has its own specific regulations regarding the dental hygienists' responsibilities. Responsibilities generally include removing deposits from teeth and providing oral health education.

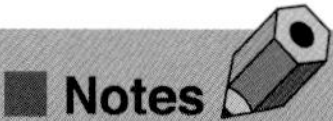

■ **Notes**

varies from state to state 州によって異なる
patient screening procedures 患者さんのスクリーニング手法
oral health condition 口腔の衛生状態 **oral cancer** 口腔癌 **inspection** 検査
dental chart 歯科カルテ **develop** 現像する **deposit** 沈着物
nutritional 栄養の **study cast** 研究用模型 **documentation** 書類作成

263-00488

What Are the Advantages of a Dental Hygiene Career?

この項では，歯科衛生士の仕事のよいところを述べています．どんなよさがあるのでしょうか？

Dental hygiene offers the following challenges and rewards：

Personal satisfaction： One of the most enjoyable aspects of a career in dental hygiene is working with people. Personal fulfillment comes from providing a valuable health care service while establishing trusting relationships with patients.

Prestige： As a result of their education and clinical training in a highly skilled discipline, dental hygienists are respected as valued members of the oral health care team.

Variety： Dental hygienists use a variety of interpersonal and clinical skills to meet the oral health needs of many different patients each day. Dental hygienists have opportunities to help special population groups such as children, the elderly and the disabled. They may also provide oral health instruction in primary and secondary schools and other settings.

Creativity： Because dental hygienists interact with such diverse population groups, they must be creative in their approach to patient management and oral health education.

Flexibility： The flexibility offered by full- and part-time employment options, as well as the availability of evening and weekend hours, enables dental hygienists to balance their career and lifestyle needs. Dental hygienists also have opportunities to work in a wide variety of settings including： private dental practices, educational and community institutions, research teams and dental corporations.

263-00488

Security： The services that dental hygienists provide are needed and valued by a large percentage of the population. There is currently a great demand for dental hygienists. Employment opportunities will be excellent well into the next century. Due to the success of preventive dentistry in reducing the incidence of oral disease, the expanding older population will retain their teeth longer, and will be even more aware of the importance of regular dental care. With the emphasis on preventive care, dentists will need to employ more dental hygienists than ever before to meet the increased demand for dental services.

Practice patterns also influence employment opportunities for Dental hygienists. With the current trend toward group practice and practice styles that stress effective and productive use of office personnel, job opportunities will continue to increase.

■ **Notes**

prestige 信望　**clinical training** 臨床実習，臨床研修　**discipline** 専門分野
variety 多様性　**population group** 集団　**the elderly** 高齢者
flexibility 柔軟性　**security** 安定性　**employment opportunities** 雇用機会
with the emphasis on ～ ～に重点をおきながら

Where Do Dental Hygienists Work?

歯科衛生士が働ける場所にはどんなところがあるのでしょうか？　雇用の機会は多いようですね．

There are many employment opportunities in the field of dental hygiene, since many dentists employ one or more dental hygienists.

Dental hygienists are in demand in general dental practices, as well as in specialty practices such as periodontics or pediatric dentistry.

263-00488

Dental hygienists are responsible for some important patient care services provided in a dental office, including removing calculus, stains and plaque from teeth, applying fluoride and pit and fissure sealants, taking and developing dental radiographs (X-rays), providing oral hygiene instructions (e.g., brushing, flossing and nutritional counseling).

Dental hygienists may also be employed to provide dental hygiene services for patients in hospitals, nursing homes and public health clinics. Depending upon the level of education and experience achieved, dental hygienists can also apply their skills and knowledge to other career activities such as teaching hygiene students in dental schools and dental hygiene education programs. Research, office management and business administration are other career options. Additionally, employment opportunities may be available with companies that market dental-related materials and equipment.

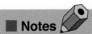

■ Notes

periodontics 歯周療法学　**pediatric dentistry** 小児歯科
pit and fissure sealant 小窩裂溝塡塞材
nutritional counseling 栄養カウンセリング
public health clinic 公立病院　**office management** 事務管理
business administration 経営管理　**market** 販売する

What Education/Training Does a Dental Hygienist Need?

歯科衛生士はどのような教育を受ける必要があるのでしょうか.

Dental hygienists receive their education through academic programs at community colleges, technical colleges, dental schools or universities. The majority of community college programs take at least two years to complete, with graduates receiving associate degrees. Receipt of this degree allows a dental hygienist to take licensure examinations (national and state or regional), become licensed and to work in a dental office. University-based dental hygiene programs may offer baccalaureate and master's degrees, which generally require at least two years of further schooling. These additional degrees may be required to embark on a career in teaching and/or research, as well as for clinical practice in school or public health programs.

Dental hygiene program admission requirements vary, depending upon the specific school. High school-level courses such as health, biology, psychology, chemistry, mathematics and speech will be beneficial in a dental hygiene career. Most programs show a preference for individuals who have completed at least one year of college. Some baccalaureate degree programs require that applicants complete two years of college prior to enrollment in the dental hygiene program. Counselors, advisors and prospective students should contact the particular dental hygiene program of interest for specific program requirements.

Dental hygiene education programs provide students with clinical education in the form of supervised patient care experiences. Additionally, these programs include courses in liberal arts (e.g., English, speech, sociology and psychology); basic sciences (e.g., anatomy, physiology, pharmacology, immunology, chemistry, microbiology and pathology); and clinical sciences (e.g., dental hygiene, radiology and dental materials). After completion of a dental hygiene program, dental hygienists can choose to pursue additional training in such areas as education, business administration, basic sciences, marketing and public health.

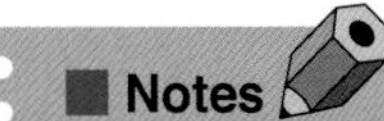

■ **Notes**

community college コミュニティ・カレッジ（2年制の短大で文系準学士・理系準学士・その他多くのプログラムを提供する）

technical college テクニカル・カレッジ（主に2年制の短大で多くのキャリア・プログラムを提供する）

263-00488

associate degree 準学士　licensure 免許下付　baccalaureate 学士号
master's degree 修士号　admission requirements 入学資格
prospective students 入学希望者　clinical education 臨床教育
patient care 患者さんのケア　liberal arts 一般教養科目　sociology 社会学
basic sciences 基礎科学　anatomy 解剖学　physiology 生理学
pharmacology 薬理学　immunology 免疫学　microbiology 微生物学
pathology 病理学　clinical science 臨床科学　radiology 放射線学

Examination and Licensure

歯科衛生士の免許を得るためには，歯科衛生士国家試験と州が認めた免許下付試験で合格点を取る必要があります．

Dental hygienists are licensed by each state to provide dental hygiene care and patient education.

Almost all states require that dental hygienists be graduates of Commission-accredited dental hygiene education programs to be eligible for state licensure. Additionally, almost all states require candidates for licensure to obtain a passing score on the National Board Dental Hygiene Examination (a comprehensive written examination) in addition to passing the state-authorized licensure examination. The state or regional examination tests candidates' clinical dental hygiene skills as well as their knowledge of dental hygiene and related subjects.

Upon receipt of their license, dental hygienists may use "R.D.H." after their names to signify recognition by the state that they are a Registered Dental Hygienist.

■ **Notes** 

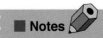

license 免許を与える　**Commission-accredited** 委員会認定の（委員会とは，

263-00488

The Commission on Dental Accreditation をさす）
eligible for ～の資格がある
the National Board Dental Hygiene Examination 歯科衛生士国家試験
state-authorized 州が認めた　**Registered Dental Hygienist** 公認歯科衛生士

●英国の場合

次に，英国の歯科衛生士事情を英国歯科衛生士会 (British Dental Hygienists' Association, BDHA) のホームページ（http://www.bdha.org.uk/）から探ってみましょう．このホームページには What can a hygienist do? というセクションがあります．ここに，英国の歯科衛生士の仕事が詳しく書かれています．

What Can a Hygienist Do?

The philosophy of dental hygiene is to prevent disease and promote health.

Some of the benefits of employing a dental hygienist：

*Patients are now aware of the highly developed expertise of a dental hygienist. As a member of the dental team the role of the dental hygienist is to motivate and treat patients to help maintain their oral health.
*The dental hygienist specialises in the prevention and treatment of oral disease focussing on periodontal health for all age groups and abilities.
*The dental hygienist also specialises in the prevention and management of dental caries.
*A dental hygienist may, following a written prescription from a registered dentist, undertake domiciliary visits for patients.
*A dental hygienist is able to complement and enhance the skilled restorative work of the dental practitioner enabling best use of clinical time.

A dental hygienist, under the written prescription of a dentist may:

263-00488

1. Monitor periodontal disease by using current indices.

2. Monitor plaque scores and provide oral hygiene advice.

3. Develop a home care plan for individual patients to maintain oral health.

4. Perform supra and subgingival scaling including comprehensive root surface debridement which may involve the use of local infiltration analgesia together with the placing of antimicrobial agents when necessary.

5. Provide a through prophylaxis which will include finishing and polishing restorations.

6. Take radiographs provided they have undergone 'core knowledge' certificate.

7. Give specific preventive advice including：

- nutritional guidance
- applying fissure sealants
- advice and use of fluoride agents
- the benefits of smoking cessation.

8. Replace crowns with temporary cement in an emergency.

9. Remove excess cement by instruments which may include rotary instruments.

10. Take impressions.

11. Administer inferior dental nerve block anaesthesia under the direct personal supervision of a registered dentist.

12. Treat patients under conscious sedation, provided a dentist remains in the room throughout the treatment.

13. Administer local infiltration anaesthesia without the direct personal supervision of a registered dentist.

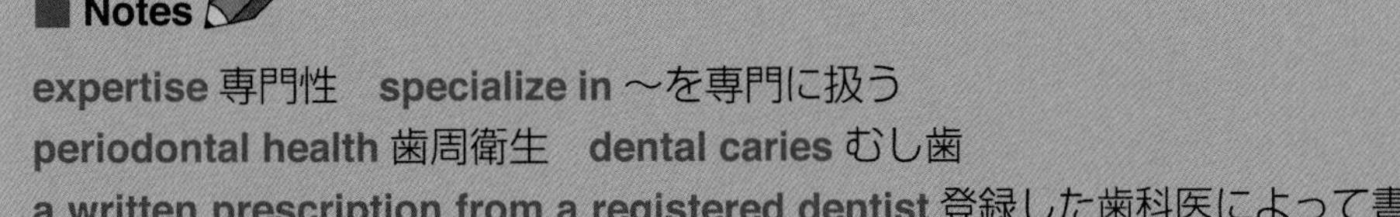

■ **Notes**

expertise 専門性　**specialize in** ～を専門に扱う
periodontal health 歯周衛生　**dental caries** むし歯
a written prescription from a registered dentist 登録した歯科医によって書かれた処方箋

263-00488

domiciliary visit 家庭訪問　**undertake** 行う
complement and enhance 補完し，強化する　**restorative work** 修復処置
dental practitioner 歯科医師　**periodontal index** 歯周指数
plaque score 歯垢指数　**supragingival** 歯肉縁上　**subgingival** 歯肉縁下
debridement 清拭　**infiltration** 浸潤　**analgesia** 無痛法
antimicrobial agent 抗菌剤　**prophylaxis** 清掃
radiograph エックス線写真　**provided** もし～ならば　**undergo** 受ける
fissure sealant 裂溝填塞材　**agent** 薬剤　**smoking cessation** 禁煙
rotary 回転式の
inferior dental nerve block anaesthesia 下歯槽神経伝達麻酔
under conscious sedation 意識下鎮静　**infiltration anaesthesia** 浸潤麻酔

Careers as a Hygienist

このセクションでは，英国における歯科衛生士の仕事が簡潔にまとめられています．

Dental hygienists can work in all sectors of dentistry, their role is twofold. They have both clinical and health promotional responsibilities. Clinically they help to treat and prevent periodontal (gum) disease by scaling and polishing teeth, applying prophylactic and antimicrobial materials, they take dental radiographs and undertake monitoring and screening procedures.

Dental hygienists are also permitted to apply topical fluorides and fissure sealants in order to reduce dental caries (tooth decay).

Their health promotional role includes motivating and encouraging individuals and groups in oral health practices including oral hygiene and diet advice.

Dental hygienists need to work with a flexible team approach; to have good communication skills and to demonstrate a high level of manual dexterity in order to

263-00488

undertake complex oral treatments.

Dental hygienist training is available at all dental schools throughout the United Kingdom. As courses vary throughout the UK please contact the Schools directly for a prospectus and details of the entry requirements.

British Dental Hygienists' Association (BDHA)
enquiries@bdha.org.uk

■ **Notes** 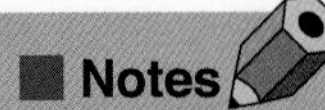

twofold 2要素からなる　**clinical** 臨床の　**health promotional** 健康増進の
periodontal disease 歯周病，歯周疾患　**prophylactic material** 予防剤
antimicrobial material 抗菌剤　**topical fluoride** フッ素歯面塗布
fissure sealant 裂溝填塞材　**diet** 食事　**manual dexterity** 手先の器用さ
prospectus 学校案内

●カナダの場合

最後に，カナダ歯科衛生士会 (The Canadian Dental Hygienists Association) のホームページ（http://www.cdha.ca/）からカナダの歯科衛生士事情をみてみましょう．

Career in Dental Hygiene

歯科衛生士になるには，何を修了し，どういった手続きが必要なのでしょうか？

In Canada, registered dental hygienists (RDHs) may pursue careers in both community and clinical practice. In order to practice, dental hygienists must complete a recognized dental hygiene program, and be registered or licensed with the appropriate provincial or territorial regulatory authorities.

263-00488

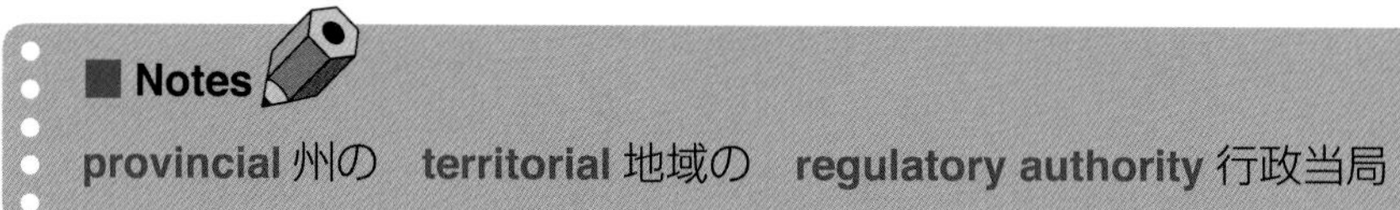

■ **Notes**
provincial 州の　**territorial** 地域の　**regulatory authority** 行政当局

Clinical Practice

歯科衛生士の臨床業務は何でしょうか？

In clinical practice, dental hygienists most often work with general practitioner dentists or specialty practice dentists. They are educated to work directly with patients to prevent and treat gum disease and tooth decay, and are trained to：

*assess tooth and gum health
*prepare individualized dental hygiene treatment plans
*refer patients to a dentist for dental treatment

As part of their clinical regime, they not only look after the cosmetic appearance of teeth and gums, but also perform complex services like scaling and root planing to treat gum infections and diseases.

Some Canadian provinces allow dental hygienists to own their own dental hygiene practice. For example, RDHs can practice independently in British Columbia, Ontario and some American states.

■ **Notes** 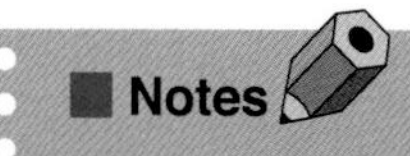
clinical practice 臨床業務　**general practitioner dentist** 一般開業歯科医師　**specialty practice dentist** 専門歯科医師　**refer patients to dentist** 患者さんに受診をすすめる

263-00488

Dialogue和訳

1　電話での予約

Warm up

患者さんから電話があったとき，受付担当者はまず，定期検診とクリーニングの予約か，緊急の手当てを必要とする問題があるのかを判断しなければなりません．救急診療の必要がないように，すべての患者さんが定期検診とクリーニングに来院することが理想です．

Dialogue

ヘルナンデスさんが定期検診とクリーニングの予約を取るために電話をかけている．受付の中西さんが電話に出ている．

中西：バレー・デンタルクリニックでございます．
ヘルナンデス：予約を取りたいのですが．
中西：定期検診でしょうか．それともすぐに手当てが必要でしょうか．
ヘルナンデス：ローラ・ヘルナンデスと申しますが，竹内先生から定期検診とクリーニングのリコールカードをいただきました．
中西：ヘルナンデスさんですね．では，先生が診察いたしますが，いつがよろしいでしょうか．
ヘルナンデス：次の金曜日はどうでしょう．
中西：はい．9時半に先生が診察，9時45分に木村がクリーニングをすることができますが．
ヘルナンデス：もう少し遅い時間にできますか．子どもたちを学校に送っていかなくてはならないので．
中西：では，10時45分ではいかがですか．
ヘルナンデス：大丈夫です．
中西：では，11月30日金曜日の10時45分にお待ちしております．
ヘルナンデス：どうもありがとうございます．

2　薬の依頼

Warm up

来院したことがないにもかかわらず，抗生物質や鎮痛剤がほしいと電話で依頼してくる人がよくいます．適切な検査や診断をせずに薬を渡すことは非常に無責任です．患者さんは必ず最初に歯科医師にみてもらわなければなりません．

Dialogue

イタリア人観光客のディリシオさんは日本に休暇で来ている．受付担当の後藤さんが，なぜ歯科医師が検査なしで薬を処方することができないかを説明している．

後藤：関東デンタルクリニックでございます．
ディリシオ：歯が痛いのですが，忙しくてクリニックに行けません．どうしたら痛みを止められますか．
後藤：はじめに歯科医師が検査して，それから一番よい治療法を決めることになります．
ディリシオ：でも，日本には2週間しかいないんですよ．それに今日は京都に行かなくちゃならないし，とても忙しいんです．
後藤：ご事情はよくわかりますが，歯科医師は検査や診断なしでは薬を処方することができないんです．
ディリシオ：そちらのクリニックに行くより仕方がないようですね．
後藤：今日の10時半でよろしければ，先生が診察できます．
ディリシオ：では10時半に行きます．
後藤：お名前と電話番号をお願いします．
ディリシオ：はい．名前はファブリッツィオ・ディリシオです．グランドハイアットの45325号室に泊まっています．
後藤：ディリシオさん，ありがとうございました．では，10時半にお待ちしています．

3　救急の予約

Warm up

診断や診療費の見積もりを電話でたずねる人がよくいます．診察をするまでは，診断をしたり治療計画を立てることはできません．

Dialogue

ムーアさんが歯痛で緊急の予約を頼んでいる．

田中：泉南国際デンタルクリニックでございます．
ムーア：歯が痛いのですが，ドクターをお願いできますか．
田中：申し訳ありませんが，先生はただいま診察中で電話に出られません．
ムーア：でも，すぐにみていただきたいのです．
田中：今日午前中でしたらみられますが，まず，どういった症状があるか説明していただけますか．
ムーア：昨日関西国際空港に着陸するときに，右上の奥歯がずきずき痛み始めたんです．
田中：何か薬は飲んでいらっしゃいますか．
ムーア：痛み止めを飲みましたが効きませんでした．ドクターはどういった処置をされるのでしょうか．
田中：最初に検査をしてエックス線写真をとる必要があります．
ムーア：歯を抜くことになりますか．
田中：鈴木先生は歯を抜かずに治療することを優先しています．最初に痛みを和らげる治療もいたします．
ムーア：私もそうしていただきたいですね．おいくらかかりますか．
田中：治療費は治療内容によります．まず，検査しなければなりません．処置の手順と費用を患者さんに説明してから治療を始めます．
ムーア：診査はおいくらですか．
田中：検査とエックス線写真で1万円です．

4　国民健康保険

Warm up

日本の健康保険をもっている外国人も多くいます．何が保険でカバーできるか，また，保険の使い方を説明することが必要になる場合もあります．

Dialogue

インドネシア出身のスハルノさんは最近日本の健康保険証を受け取った．受付担当の竹田さんに治療についてたずねている．

スハルノ：日本の健康保険証があるのですが，使えますか．
竹田：はい，もちろんです．
スハルノ：保険で治療全部の支払いができるのですか．
竹田：いいえ．費用の3割を患者さんが支払うことになります．
スハルノ：ドクターは治療にいくらかかるか教えてくださいますか．
竹田：もちろんです．何かする前には必ず患者さんの同意を取ります．もし何か質問がある場合は必ず先生にたずねてください．
スハルノ：クラウンに保険はききますか．
竹田：はい，保険でカバーできますが，ポーセレンクラウンにはききません．
スハルノ：白い色の充填物はどうですか．
竹田：コンポジットレジンの充填には使えます．
スハルノ：コンポジットレジンってなんですか．
竹田：コンポジットレジンというのはプラスチックとガラス半々でできていて，本物の歯のようにみえるものです．
スハルノ：私はそれがいいです．

5　患者さんに症状を説明してもらう

Warm up

急患は歯科医師のスケジュールが詰まっているときに来院することもあります．歯科医師の時間を節約するために，歯科衛生士は患者さんに症状を説明してもらい，診察前に歯科医師に伝えることができます．

Dialogue

マースデンさんは歯痛の治療のため来院した．歯科衛生士の佐藤さんは歯科医師に伝えるため症状についていくつか質問をしている．

佐藤：歯が痛いそうですね．
マースデン：ええ．痛くて死にそうです．
佐藤：村田先生にあなたの症状について報告できるよう2，3質問させていただきます．
マースデン：どうぞ．
佐藤：まず，どの歯が痛みますか．
マースデン：奥の右下です．
佐藤：正確にどの歯かわかりますか．
マースデン：はっきりわからないんです．
佐藤：いつから痛み始めましたか．
マースデン：数週間前から気になっていたんですが，昨日から本当に悪くなりました．
佐藤：熱いものや冷たいものでしみますか．
マースデン：最初は冷たいものだけしみたんですが，いまでは熱いものを飲むとずきずき痛むんです．
佐藤：最近歯科治療を受けられましたか．
マースデン：2～3カ月前に奥から2番目の歯にクラウンをかぶせてもらいましたが，むし歯がとても深いと先生にいわれました．
佐藤：その歯が問題かもしれませんね．
マースデン：ドクターはどういうことをされるんでしょうか．
佐藤：まず，エックス線写真を撮って診断をします．それからどういう治療をするか説明することになります．
マースデン：わかりました．
佐藤：甘いものはどうですか．痛みが起こりますか．
マースデン：いえ，それほどでもありません．
佐藤：かむときは痛みますか．
マースデン：はい．この数日は左側だけでかんでいます．
佐藤：村田先生に報告いたします．先生はもうすぐ参ります．
マースデン：どうもありがとうございます．

6　病歴をたずねる

Warm up

患者さんに病歴をたずねるよう歯科医師から依頼があるかもしれません．患者さんがいったことは書き留めて歯科医師に渡さなければなりません．歯科衛生士が理解できない医学的問題は歯科医師に任せるべきです．

Dialogue

メータさんは初診で来院した．歯科衛生士の阿部さんが歯科医師による診察の前に病歴をたずねている．

阿部：清水先生から病歴を記録するようにいわれました．
メータ：どうしてそれが必要なのですか．ただ歯を検査してほしいだけですよ．
阿部：体の状態が歯や歯ぐきに影響を与えることもあるんですよ．
メータ：本当ですか？
阿部：はい．それに，医師が薬を処方する前にはアレルギーや医学的問題があるかどうか知っておかなければなりません．
メータ：わかりました．
阿部：いままでに重い病気になったことはありますか．
メータ：20年前に皮膚癌で治療を受けましたが，再発はいまのところありません．
阿部：わかりました．何か薬は飲んでいますか．
メータ：頭痛のときタイレノールを飲むことはあります．
阿部：薬や歯科の麻酔にアレルギーはありますか．
メータ：ええ．ペニシリンにアレルギーがあります．抗生物質が必要なら何を処方してくださるのでしょうか．
阿部：私にはわかりかねますので，先生とお話なさってください．このことはカルテに書いておきますので先生もたずねられるはずです．
メータ：ありがとうございます．
阿部：クラウンや根管治療などの大きな歯科治療は受けたことがおありですか．
メータ：いえ．歯を詰めただけです．

263-00488

阿部：親知らずは抜きましたか．
メータ：ええ．10年前に4本全部抜きました．
阿部：わかりました．では清水先生に報告いたします．
メータ：ありがとうございます．

7　歯周病

Part Ⅰ

Warm up

歯科衛生士は歯周病について患者さんに説明するように歯科医師から頼まれることがよくあります．このような場合，歯や歯ぐきがどのようになっているか絵を見せながら説明すると患者さんは理解しやすいものです．

Dialogue

歯科衛生士の藤田さんは，歯周病について患者さんのガルシアさんに説明するように歯科医師から依頼された．

藤田：田中先生から歯周病の説明をするようにといわれました．
ガルシア：なんだか深刻に聞こえますね．そんなに悪くなってますか．
藤田：ガルシアさんの場合はまだ初期なのでよい状態に戻すことは可能です．でも，もし治療しないと歯周病が原因で歯を失うことにもなります．
ガルシア：歯は失いたくないですね．
藤田：歯周病の説明をするために歯の絵を描いてみますね．
ガルシア：ありがとうございます．そうしていただくと助かります．
藤田：この絵は歯と歯ぐきの様子を示しています．歯の根は，歯ぐきの上に現れている歯の部分と同じぐらいの大きさをしています．
ガルシア：それは知りませんでした．
藤田：歯はまわりの歯ぐきと骨で支えられているのです．
ガルシア：はい．
藤田：歯と歯ぐきの間には3mmぐらいの深さの歯周ポケットがあります．食べ物や細菌，カルシウム沈着物がこのポケットに入ると，歯根についている組織を破壊します．
ガルシア：それはこわいですね．
藤田：そうです．それが歯周病の原因です．

Part Ⅱ

Warm up

Part Ⅰの会話の続きです．

Dialogue

歯科衛生士がどのようにして歯周病を治療するか説明している．

ガルシア：先生はどのように私の歯周病を治療されるのですか．
藤田：最初の治療は私がこのスケーラーのような特別の器具を使って行います．
ガルシア：それは何ですか．
藤田：これは歯ぐきの上と下の両方についた歯垢やカルシウム沈着物を取り除く器具です．
ガルシア：それはなんの役に立つんですか．
藤田：こうすることで歯の周りの組織が健康になり，歯周病を治すことができるのです．
ガルシア：もし，その治療をしなかったら？
藤田：細菌が歯を支えている組織を破壊し続けます．
ガルシア：こわいですね．
藤田：そのとおりです．この絵のように骨は破壊され，歯もぐらついてきます．
ガルシア：それは嫌ですね．

8　妊娠

Warm up

妊娠に関連したホルモンが歯ぐきの腫れや不快感を引き起こすことがよくあります．これは歯周病ではありませんが，妊娠中は口腔を健康に保つ必要があります．

Dialogue

歯科衛生士の大谷さんが患者さんのジェンセンさんに，妊娠が口腔衛生にどのように影響するかを説明している．

ジェンセン：私は妊娠しているのですが，歯のクリーニングをしても大丈夫ですか．
大谷：歯のクリーニングをするのは全く問題ありません．それどころか，妊娠中に口腔を健康に保つことはとても大切なのですよ．
ジェンセン：実を言えば，最近歯ぐきがちょっと不快な感じなんです．
大谷：それは，妊娠中よくあることです．
ジェンセン：どうしてですか．
大谷：妊娠に関連するホルモンが歯ぐきの腫れを引き起こすのです．
ジェンセン：それは知りませんでした．何か困ったことになりますか．
大谷：深刻ではありませんが，歯をクリーニングしたら気持ちよくなりますよ．
ジェンセン：エックス線写真は必要ですか．
大谷：深刻な状態がない限り，歯科医師は妊娠中の患者さんのエックス線写真を撮ることはしません．
ジェンセン：それはよかったです．ではなるべく早く予約をお願いします．

9　なぜクリーニングが必要か

Warm up

歯科衛生士の重要な役目の一つは患者さんを教育することです．患者さんが治療の内容と理由を理解すれば，治療への満足度も高まり，ひいては歯科診療所に再来院する可能性も高くなります．

Dialogue

歯科衛生士の吉田さんが患者さんのベレスフォードさんにクリーニングの必要性を説明している．

ベレスフォード：なぜ，クリーニングが必要なんですか．僕は毎日歯を磨いていますよ．
吉田：私たちがするクリーニングは歯肉縁下の歯石や，歯垢，歯のステインを取り除くものです．
ベレスフォード：歯ブラシでできないんですか．
吉田：歯ブラシで落とすことのできない歯石やカルシウム沈着物を落とす特別な器具を使います．

ベレスフォード：歯石ってなんですか.
吉田：長期間の間に歯の表面に発生するカルシウム沈着物です．とても硬いものなので歯ブラシでは取れません.
ベレスフォード：もし，クリーニングをしてもらっても，毎日ブラッシングする必要はあるのですか.
吉田：はい．歯垢を取るために毎日ブラッシングとフロスをするのはとても大切です.
ベレスフォード：歯垢とは？
吉田：細菌と食べかすからできた薄い膜で，歯の表面と歯肉縁下にできます.
ベレスフォード：説明ありがとうございます.
吉田：では，イスを倒してクリーニングを始めます.
ベレスフォード：お願いします.

10　インフォームドコンセント

Part Ⅰ

Warm up

いかなる医療行為の前にも，患者さんが自分の治療について理解していることが大切です．患者さんはその治療がなぜ，どのように行われ，費用がいくらかかるかを理解しなければなりません．これはインフォームドコンセントとよばれています．米国では，歯科医師が忙しいため，歯科衛生士が代わってこの説明をすることがよくあります.

Dialogue

歯科衛生士の立木さんが香港のビジネスマン，チョウさんに治療と費用の説明をしている.

立木：チョウさん，こんにちは．松井先生から治療計画を説明するようにいわれましたが，よろしいでしょうか.
チョウ：ありがとうございます．お願いします.
立木：松井先生が診察したところ，治療の必要なむし歯が2つ見つかりました.
チョウ：ええ．先生から聞きました.
立木：2つとも左の下側です.
チョウ：はい，1本は痛みがあります.
立木：その歯は根管治療が必要です.
チョウ：根管治療？　なんだか痛そうですね.
立木：大丈夫です．松井先生はとても丁寧ですから．麻酔もしますし，処置はぜんぜん痛くありません.
チョウ：根管治療とは何か説明していただけますか.
立木：はい．歯の絵を描いて説明しましょう.
チョウ：ありがとうございます.
立木：これがあなたの歯です．いいですか？（立木さんが絵を描く）　これは小臼歯です．そこにむし歯があって根に影響を与えているわけです.
チョウ：なるほど.
立木：だから，痛みがあるのです．松井先生は麻酔でその歯の感覚を麻痺させます．よろしいですか？
チョウ：そうしていただけるとありがたいです.
立木：それから，歯の根管から感染した組織を取り除きます．（立木さんが根管の絵を指し示す）
チョウ：そうすると，組織は取り除かれるのですね.
立木：そのとおりです.
チョウ：時間はどのくらいかかりますか.
立木：2，3分しかかかりません．それから，先生が歯の根管に充填物をいれます.
チョウ：その歯は死んだことになるんですか.
立木：はい．もう歯の中には神経がなくなるわけですから.
チョウ：えーっ！それは困ったなあ.
立木：でも，そんなに大変な問題でもありません．一生その歯を失わずに，普通に使えますから.
チョウ：まあ，歯を失ってしまうよりいいでしょうね.

Part Ⅱ

Warm up

Part Ⅰの会話の続きです.

Dialogue

歯科衛生士が，根管治療の後どのように歯が修復されるか，また費用がどれだけかかるかを説明している.

チョウ：根管治療が終わった後は，どういうことをするんですか.
立木：先生が歯の前処置をし，型を取ります.
チョウ：それはどのくらい時間がかかるんですか.
立木：全部で90分ぐらいですね．松井先生が仮のクラウンをかぶせます.
チョウ：本当のクラウンはいつかぶせてもらえるのですか.
立木：2週間でできます.
チョウ：もう1つのむし歯はどうなりますか.
立木：そちらのほうはもっと小さいですね．この絵をご覧になってください．クラウンをかぶせるために来院されたときに先生が充填をします.
チョウ：水銀の詰め物は嫌なのですが.
立木：先生は水銀を使った充填はしません.
チョウ：そうですか．よかった.
立木：歯と同じ色のコンポジットレジンを使うことになります.
チョウ：私もそれがいいですね．全部で費用はいくらかかりますか.
立木：今日は検査とエックス線写真で8,000円です．根管治療は30,000円,クラウンは110,000円です．ここに値段を全部お書きします.
チョウ：そうしていただけると助かります．充填はおいくらですか.
立木：20,000円でできます．クリーニングもなさったほうがいいですね．もしお望みでしたら今日できますよ．8,000円です.
チョウ：それをしていただきたいですね.
立木：この絵のコピーは私たちの記録のためにとっておきますので，原画をお渡しします.
チョウ：ありがとうございます．これを全部妻に説明しなければなりません.
立木：もし私がお答えできない質問が

263-00488

ありましたら,松井先生が喜んで対応させていただきます.
チョウ:ありがとうございます.

11　シーラント

Part Ⅰ

Warm up

子どもの親から，シーラントに関しての質問を受けることがあります．これは大切な治療であり永久臼歯に深い溝のある子どもすべてにすすめられるものです．もちろん，親にだけでなく子どもにもすべて説明をしなければなりません．治療説明のパンフレットを親に渡すのもいいでしょう．

Dialogue

鈴木先生はボビー・ミラーにシーラントをすすめた．歯科衛生士の児島さんがなぜシーラントが必要なのかをボビーの母親に説明している．

児島:鈴木先生が，ボビー君にはシーラントが必要だといっています．
ミラー:どうして必要なのですか．
児島:説明しますので，このパンフレットをご覧ください．
ミラー:ありがとうございます．
児島:シーラントというのは白いプラスチックの薄い層で，臼歯の溝に埋めてむし歯を予防するものです．
ミラー:どのように予防の助けになるのですか．
児島:永久臼歯は深い溝があって，そこから簡単にむし歯になりやすいのです．
ミラー:私が子どものときはシーラントをしなかったですけれど．
児島:もしされていたら役に立っていたはずです．
ミラー:どうしてですか．
児島:このエックス線写真をご覧ください．お母さんの臼歯8本全部に充填物かクラウンがありますね．
ミラー:ボビーには，私のような歯になってほしくありません．

Part Ⅱ

Warm up

Part Ⅰの会話の続きです．子どもに説明するときは，怖がらせないように簡単な言葉を使うことが大事です．

Dialogue

児島さんがどのようにしてシーラントを行うか患者さんのボビーに説明している．

ボビー:シーラントは難しいの？
児島:とっても簡単よ．鈴木先生がどういうことをするのかみせてあげましょう．
ボビー:痛い？
児島:全然嫌な感じなんてしないのよ．ボビー君の手をみせてくれる？それで説明してあげるから．
ボビー:いいよ．
児島:爪の上にシーラントをする真似をしてみましょう．
ボビー:おもしろそう．
児島:鈴木先生が電動歯ブラシに歯磨きをつけてこういうふうにボビー君の歯を磨いてくれるのよ．
ボビー:くすぐったーい．
児島:それからスプレーの水で歯磨きを洗い流すの．こういうふうにね．
ボビー:手にもってる掃除機みたいなのは何？
児島:これは口の中の掃除機よ．爪にスプレーした水をきれいにするために使うの．
ボビー:おもしろいね．
児島:じゃあ，この白いプラスチックの液を爪にかけましょう．鈴木先生がボビー君の歯にかけるみたいに．
ボビー:たのしいね．
児島:次はちょっとの間だけプラスチックに光をあてましょう．この光でプラスチックが硬くなるのよ．
ボビー:わー！コンタクトレンズみたい．
児島:爪からは簡単に削り落とせるけれど，鈴木先生が歯にかけるのは何年間ももつのよ．
ボビー:すごいね．

12　フッ素治療

Warm up

子どもの治療を始める前には，どういう医療行為がなぜ行われるかを親に知らせなければなりません．これは，充塡，抜歯，そしてフッ素治療であっても行わなければなりません．

Dialogue

歯科衛生士の野中さんがウッズさんに，彼女の息子の歯になぜフッ素治療が必要なのか説明している．

ウッズ:フッ素治療とは何ですか．
野中:歯を完全にクリーニングした後，高濃度のフッ素溶液を入れたプラスチックのトレーをお子さんの口の中に4分間入れるのです．
ウッズ:なぜ，この治療をするのですか．
野中:フッ素イオンが歯の表面に浸透して，エナメル質をむし歯に対して抵抗力のあるものにするのです．
ウッズ:でも，フッ素入り歯磨きでいつも歯を磨いてやっていますが，それで十分じゃないのですか．
野中:フッ素入り歯磨きを使うのは大切です．特に子どもには．
ウッズ:では，なぜここでフッ素治療をするんですか．
野中:ここで私たちがする治療は高濃度のフッ素を使います．歯磨きに入っているフッ素よりもっと効果的なのです．
ウッズ:フッ素の錠剤を毎日与えていますけれど，それでもフッ素治療は必要なのですか．
野中:フッ素の錠剤は歯にとてもいいですが，フッ素治療はそれでも必要です．2つはそれぞれ違うものですから．
ウッズ:どう違うのですか．
野中:お母さんが与えていらっしゃる錠剤の中のフッ素は，お子さんのあごが発達していく過程で歯の中に結合して取り込まれていくものです．
ウッズ:ここでするフッ素治療とどう違うのですか．
野中:ここでする治療はフッ素イオンを，すでに生えている歯のエナメル質の表面層の中に入れるものです．
ウッズ:フッ素治療はどのくらいの頻度でしなければなりませんか．
野中:定期検診にこられる6カ月ごと

にしたほうがいいです．
ウッズ：いろいろ説明をありがとうございました．

13　子どものための歯ブラシ指導

Warm up

子どもを治療する際の歯科衛生士の大切な役目の一つとして，歯科医師への恐怖感をなくすことが挙げられます．小さな子どもの歯をクリーニングするときは，どういうことをするのか全部説明し，シリンジ以外の器具をすべてみせるようにします．鏡を渡して，診療中何をしているのかみえるようにしてあげるのもいいでしょう．子どもは何をされているか実際にみることができるとリラックスするものです．子どもでも理解できる言葉だけをつかうことが大切です．また，子どものブラッシングを日々管理するのは親の役目ですから，子どもに歯ブラシ指導をしている間，親にも立ち会ってもらうとよいでしょう．

Dialogue

歯科衛生士の谷口さんが7歳のジェイニーに歯ブラシ指導をしている．

ジェイニー：あなたは誰？
谷口：私は歯の看護師よ．
ジェイニー：私に何するの？
谷口：歯の磨き方をみせてあげるのよ．
ジェイニー：痛い？
谷口：いいえ．鏡をみてくれる？
ジェイニー：いいよ．
谷口：はじめに歯の外側を磨くのよ．こういうふうにね．自分でやってみてくれる？
ジェイニー：うん．これでいい？
谷口：上手ね．じゃあ，1つの歯を10回ずつ磨きながら，こういうふうに歯の外側をぐるっと全部回っていって．
ジェイニー：くすぐったい．
谷口：そしたら，歯の内側も同じようにブラシしてね．
ジェイニー：おもしろいね．
谷口：今度は，かみ合うところも．
ジェイニー：楽しいね．
谷口：上の歯も同じようにしてちょうだい．舌をブラシするのも忘れないで．
ジェイニー：はい．
谷口：ちゃんと磨けているかおかあさんにも確かめてもらってね．
ジェイニー：いつも手伝ってもらってるよ．
谷口：それはよかった．歯ブラシが終わったら，お母さんにフロスしてもらうのよ．

14　大人のための歯ブラシ指導

Warm up

患者さんに歯ブラシ指導をするときは，何をしているかみえるように，鏡を持たせることが大切です．患者さんは，ブラッシングの方法と，その理由について理解しなければなりません．

Dialogue

歯科衛生士の松田さんが，御殿場に住んでいる交換留学生のコーエンさんに歯ブラシ指導をしています．

コーエン：本当に1日3回歯磨きをする必要があるのですか．
松田：歯垢は2～3時間で歯につきます．定期的に歯垢を取り除かないとむし歯や歯周病，口臭の原因になります．
コーエン：デンタルリンスを使っていますが，それでは十分じゃないのですか．
松田：はい．デンタルリンスだけでは十分ではありません．ブラッシングすることで歯の表面のねばねばした歯垢を取り除けますし，フロスは歯と歯の間の歯垢を取り除きます．
コーエン：ブラッシングの方法をみせていただけますか．
松田：承知しました．私がおみせする間，この鏡を持ってご覧になっていてください．
コーエン：はい．
松田：歯ブラシの毛を歯に対してこのように45度の角度にもっていきます．
コーエン：それだと歯ぐきを傷めませんか？
松田：いいえ，正しいタイプの歯ブラシと適切なテクニックを使えば，大丈夫です．歯ぐきを傷つけないよう，やわらかい毛の歯ブラシを使ってください．
コーエン：わかりました．
松田：一度に2～3回円を描くように磨いてください．それからブラシをこのように前に倒して2～3回磨いてください．
コーエン：これだとずいぶん時間がかかりますね．
松田：それほどでもありません．全部磨き終わるのに3分ぐらいでできるはずです．
コーエン：そんなに長くはないですね．
松田：歯の外側を磨いた後は，舌に面している内側を磨いてください．
コーエン：いままでそんなことしたことがなかったです．
松田：だから，歯にたくさん歯垢がたまっているのです．最後に咬合面も磨いてください．
コーエン：それだけですか．
松田：いえ，まだです．上の歯も同じようにしてください．
コーエン：それでおしまいですか．
松田：もう一つあります．舌もブラッシングするべきです．
コーエン：なぜですか．そんなこといままでしたことがありませんが．
松田：舌の表面に蓄積する細菌は口臭の原因になります．
コーエン：それは困ります．
松田：1日に3回歯を磨き，毎日少なくとも1回全部の歯をフロスしてください．
コーエン：町で一番歯がきれいな人になりそう．
松田：そうなるといいですね．

15　患者さんへの診察後の指示

Part Ⅰ

Warm up

治療が終わった後，患者さんに診察後の指示を与えるのは歯科衛生士や歯科助手の責任になることがよくあります．これは忘れてしまいがちですが，そうすることで患者さんからは非常に感謝されるものです．

263-00488

Dialogue

カーンさんはクリーニングと下顎第二大臼歯にコンポジットレジン充填を受けたところです．歯科衛生士の松原さんが診察後の指示を与えています．

松原：山平先生から診察後の指示をするようにいわれました．
カーン：しびれはどのくらいでなくなりますか．
松原：通常，2〜3時間ぐらいです．
カーン：もっと早くなるように何か自分でできることはありますか．
松原：あごをやさしくマッサージしてもいいですが，ご心配はいりません．麻酔は自然にきれますから．
カーン：その歯で食べられるようになるまで，1日待たなければなりませんか．
松原：アマルガム充填の場合はそうですが，コンポジットレジンは歯に入れた後すぐ固まります．
カーン：それはよかった．
松原：麻酔がきれたらすぐかめますよ．
カーン：でも，いまおなかがすいているのですが．
松原：かむ必要のあるものは何も食べないようにしてください．気づかずに，唇や舌をかんでしまうことがありますから．
カーン：ジュースなどは飲んでいいですか．
松原：飲むのは大丈夫ですし，ヨーグルトやスープのようなかむ必要のないものも食べて大丈夫です．

Part Ⅱ

Warm up

Part Ⅰの会話の続きです．

Dialogue

歯科衛生士の松原さんが診療後の指示をカーンさんに与えています．

松原：麻酔がきれる前にあまり熱いものは飲まないように注意してください．
カーン：それはどうしてですか．
松原：コーヒーのような熱い飲みものは唇をやけどするおそれがありますが，唇が麻痺していると気がつかないのです．
カーン：クリーニングのせいで歯ぐきが痛む場合はどうしたらいいでしょうか．
松原：2年間クリーニングされていなかったので，明日は歯ぐきや歯が少し過敏になっているかもしれません．
カーン：はい，それはそうでしょうね．
松原：やわらかい毛の歯ブラシで磨いてください．歯ぐきにはそっとやさしくあてるように．
カーン：痛い場合，タイレノールを飲んでもいいですか．
松原：もし，必要と思われるなら大丈夫です．それから，冷たいもので歯が少ししみるかもしれません．
カーン：なぜですか．
松原：歯肉ラインに近い部分のカルシウム沈着物が取り除かれたので，歯が口の中の液体や飲み物にさらされ過敏になるわけです．
カーン：それはどのくらい続くのでしょうか．
松原：普通2〜3日でなくなります．
カーン：しみるのを防ぐためにできることはありますか．
松原：一番よいのは知覚過敏用歯磨きを使って磨くことですね．
カーン：教えてくださってありがとうございました．

16　治療後

Warm up

治療が完了した後，受付担当がしなければならない重要なことが三つあります．歯科医師が処方した薬を患者さんに渡すこと，次の予約を取ること，そして治療費を徴収することです．

Dialogue

ライトさんはクラウンのための歯の形成と印象をとって今回のアポイントを終えた．受付担当の北村さんが彼女と話している．

北村：今日の治療はいかがでしたか．
ライト：実際には，思ったほど痛くなかったですね．
北村：それはよかったです．先生からこのお薬をお渡しするようにとのことです．
ライト：ありがとうございます．それは何ですか．
北村：痛み止めのボルタレンです．もし必要ならば，5〜6時間おきに1錠か2錠お飲みください．
ライト：問題がなくても飲む必要があるのですか．
北村：いいえ，必要だと思われるときだけ飲んでください．
ライト：キム先生はとても丁寧だったので，薬を飲む必要はないと思いますが．でも，いただいておきます．ありがとうございます．
北村：どういたしまして．次の予約はクラウンを入れるために2週間後にしましょう．4月7日の木曜日はだいじょうぶですか．
ライト：ええ，けっこうです．9時に来てもいいですか．
北村：その時間はもう予約が入っています．10時でもよろしいでしょうか．
ライト：それでも大丈夫です．どのくらいの時間がかかりますか．
北村：30分ぐらいです．
ライト：新しいクラウンを入れていただくのが楽しみです．
北村：きっとご満足いただけると思います．今日の治療費は2万円です．
ライト：クレジットカードで支払ってもいいですか．
北村：もちろんです．

17　米国の歯科診療所訪問

Part Ⅰ

Warm up

日本や外国の歯科診療所を訪問することはとても教育的効果があります．

Dialogue

札幌の歯科衛生士である竹内順子さんが，サンフランシスコのデンタルクリニックを訪問し，クリニックマネジャーのメリー・ボイドさんと話をしている．

順子：ボイドさん，こちらのクリニックに招待していただきありがとうございます.

メリー：こんにちは．順子さん，おいでいただいてうれしいです．メリーとよんでください.

順子： 日本から来ていますので，人をファーストネームでよぶのには慣れていないんです.

メリー：このクリニックでは，患者さんも含めてみんなお互いをファーストネームでよぶんです．そのほうが親しみがもてるでしょう.

順子：大きな歯科診療所ですね．ここでは何人の方が働いていらっしゃるのですか.

メリー：ここはチーム医療です．歯科医師が5人とスタッフが23人います.

順子：うわ，すごい．たくさんの方々をマネージしていらっしゃるのですね．まるで会社を経営しているみたいですね.

メリー：実際に会社なんですよ．大きな歯科診療所は会社組織になっているところが多いのです.

順子：一つの歯科診療所にどうしてそんなにたくさんの歯科医師がいるのですか.

メリー：2人が一般歯科医，1人が小児歯科医，1人が補綴歯科医，1人が歯周病専門医です.

順子：日本では歯科医師はひとりでなんでもこなすのが当然と思われています．専門医はほとんどいません.

メリー：デカスロンの歯科みたいですね．米国では，歯科医師が難しいケースを専門医にまわすことがよくあります．患者さんができる限り最良の治療を受けられるようにです.

順子：それはいい考えですね.

Part Ⅱ

Warm up

Part Ⅰの会話の続きです.

Dialogue

オフィスマネジャーのメリー・ボイドが竹内順子さんに歯科診療所を案内している.

順子：なぜ，そんなに多くのスタッフが必要なのですか.

メリー：3人がフロントで働いています．歯科衛生士が10人，歯科助手が8人，常勤で消毒担当をしているのが2人います.

順子：私が働いている歯科診療所では，私が全部することになっています.

メリー：それじゃあ，デカスロンの歯科衛生士版ね.

順子：することがいっぱいあって…….ここでは国民健康保険が使えるのですか.

メリー：米国には国民健康保険というのはないんです．ほとんどの患者さんは民間保険会社の保険をもっています.

順子：歯科衛生士の部屋を一つみせていただけますか.

メリー：もちろんです．ここはジョンの部屋です.

順子：日本では歯科衛生士は全員女性です.

メリー：いま米国では男性の歯科衛生士もたくさんいますよ.

順子：歯科衛生士に助手がいるのはなぜですか.

メリー：普通，歯科衛生士は一人で仕事をしますが，ルートプレーニングのような難しいケースだと助手がつきます.

順子：彼は歯科衛生士なのに，麻酔をしているのはなぜですか.

メリー：カリフォルニアの歯科衛生士はトレーニングを受けて局部麻酔を行うことができるのです.

順子：それは責任が重いですね.

メリー：歯科衛生士は非常に尊敬される職業です.

263-00488

Reading解答

p.7

A1 Yes.

A2 Please give your child a nutritious foods (Example).

A3 Milk, fresh fruits, vegetables etc (Example).

p.13

A1 I use a soft-bristle and small-size toothbrush (Example).

A2 No, I have never used it (Example).

A3 It will cause teeth sensitivity and gums injury.

p.19

A1 37 (Three-seven)

A2 13 (One-three)

A3 81 (Eight-one)

p.23

A1 Yes

A2 More than 108 million.

A3 Lack of dental insurance.

p.31

A1 No, you should pick it up by the crown.

A2 No, it is not.

A3 One of the methods is wearing a mouthguard.

p.47

A1 The risks of lung cancer, heart disease and cerebral stroke increase.

A2 The risks of oral cancer and periodontal disease increase.

A3 The smoking rates are 47% in males and 11% in felames (2003).

p.53

A1 Poor oral hygiene causes pregnancy gingivitis.

A2 No, usually it returns to normal gums.

A3 Thorough tooth brushing and flossing.

p.59

A1 Because goals have to be established on the basis of local situations.

A2 No, there is not.

A3 Smoking, poor oral hygiene, stress and some systemic diseases.

p.71

A1 The process by which fully informed patients can participate in choices about their dental care.

A2 It is mentioned above 1 to 6.

A3 Provide additional information about dental treatment.

p.86

A1 Yes, it is.

A2 Fluoride mouthrinse, direct fluoride application, and fluoride toothpaste.

A3 Fluoridated water, fluoridated foods, and fluoride supplements.

p.93

A1 Yes.

A2 It causes tooth decays.

A3 To give a healthy food (Example).

p.99

A1 Twice, in the morning and at night (Example).

A2 Dentists and dental hygienists.

A3 Every 2 to 3 months.

p.109

A1 Be careful not to bite or burn your tongue, cheeks, or lips while you are numb.

A2 Yes.

A3 Call the dentist as soon as possible.

p.125

A1 The roles are prevention of dental diseases, health education and assistance for dental treatment.

A2 About 143,000 dental hygienists are working (2020).

A3 Yes, I am (Example).

263-00488

歯科用頻出単語296（p.136～141）出典サイト

1. The American Dental Hygienists' Association
http://www.adha.org/

2. National Center for Biotechnology Information (paper abstract)
http://www.ncbi.nlm.nih.gov/

(1) Educational needs and employment status of Scottish dental nurses. (Ross MK, Ibbetson RJ, Rennie JS, 2005)
http://www.ncbi.nlm.nih.gov/sites/entrez?Db=pubmed&Cmd=ShowDetailView&TermToSearch=17128241&ordinalpos=1&itool=EntrezSystem2.PEntrez.Pubmed.Pubmed_ResultsPanel.Pubmed_RVDocSum

(2) Brushing with and without dentifrice on gingival abrasion. (Versteeg PA, Timmerman MF, Piscaer M, Van der Velden U, Van der Weijden GA, 2005)
http://www.ncbi.nlm.nih.gov/sites/entrez?Db=pubmed&Cmd=ShowDetailView&TermToSearch=15691345&ordinalpos=3&itool=EntrezSystem2.PEntrez.Pubmed.Pubmed_ResultsPanel.Pubmed_RVDocSum

(3) Routine scale and polish for periodontal health in adults. (Beirne P, Forgie A, Worthington HV, Clarkson JE, 2005)
http://www.ncbi.nlm.nih.gov/sites/entrez?Db=pubmed&Cmd=ShowDetailView&TermToSearch=15674957&ordinalpos=3&itool=EntrezSystem2.PEntrez.Pubmed.Pubmed_ResultsPanel.Pubmed_RVDocSum

(4) The role of dental hygienists in oral health prevention. (Ohrn K, 2004)
http://www.ncbi.nlm.nih.gov/sites/entrez?Db=pubmed&Cmd=ShowDetailView&TermToSearch=15646586&ordinalpos=10&itool=EntrezSystem2.PEntrez.Pubmed.Pubmed_ResultsPanel.Pubmed_RVDocSum

(5) What drives the practice? (Levin RP, 2004)
http://www.ncbi.nlm.nih.gov/sites/entrez?Db=pubmed&Cmd=ShowDetailView&TermToSearch=15643767&ordinalpos=91&itool=EntrezSystem2.PEntrez.Pubmed.Pubmed_ResultsPanel.Pubmed_RVDocSum

(6) Self-perceived oral function elderly residents in a suburban area of Stockholm, Sweden. (Andersson K, Gustafsson A, Buhlin K, 2004)
http://www.ncbi.nlm.nih.gov/sites/entrez

(7) Oral health in Syria. (Beiruti N, van Palenstein Helderman WH, 2004)
http://www.ncbi.nlm.nih.gov/sites/entrez?Db=pubmed&Cmd=ShowDetailView&TermToSearch=15631101&ordinalpos=2&itool=EntrezSystem2.PEntrez.Pubmed.Pubmed_ResultsPanel.Pubmed_RVDocSum

(8) The role of dental therapists working in four personal dental service pilots: type of patients seen, work undertaken and cost-effectiveness within the context of the dental practice. (Harris R, Burnside G, 2004)
http://www.ncbi.nlm.nih.gov/sites/entrez

(9) A baseline study of the demographics of the oral health workforce in rural and remote Western Australia. (Kruger E, Tennant M, 2004)
http://www.ncbi.nlm.nih.gov/sites/entrez

(10) Occlusal sealant success over ten years in a private practice: comparing longevity of sealants placed by dentists, hygienists, and assistants. (Folke BD, Walton JL, Feigal RJ, 2004)
http://www.ncbi.nlm.nih.gov/sites/entrez

(11) Oral hygiene reduces respiratory infections in elderly bed-bound nursing home patients. (Yoneyama T, Hashimoto K, Fukuda H, Ishida M, Arai H, Sekizawa K, Yamaya M, Sasaki H, 1996)
http://www.ncbi.nlm.nih.gov/sites/entrez?Db=

263-00488

pubmed&Cmd=ShowDetailView&TermToSearch=15374188&ordinalpos=3&itool=EntrezSystem2.PEntrez.Pubmed.Pubmed_ResultsPanel.Pubmed_RVDocSum

(12) Plaque removal by professional electric toothbrushing compared with professional polishing. (Van der Weijden GA, Timmerman MF, Piscaer M, Ijzerman Y, Van der Velden U, 2004)
http://www.ncbi.nlm.nih.gov/sites/entrez?Db=pubmed&Cmd=ShowDetailView&TermToSearch=15367196&ordinalpos=2&itool=EntrezSystem2.PEntrez.Pubmed.Pubmed_ResultsPanel.Pubmed_RVDocSum

(13) Attitudes to independent dental hygiene practice: dentists and dental hygienists in Ontario. (Adams TL, 2004)
http://www.ncbi.nlm.nih.gov/sites/entrez?Db=pubmed&Cmd=ShowDetailView&TermToSearch=15363213&ordinalpos=3&itool=EntrezSystem2.PEntrez.Pubmed.Pubmed_ResultsPanel.Pubmed_RVDocSum

(14) Survey of hepatitis B and C in students of faculty of dentistry and dental hygienist school. (Nagao Y, Chibo I, Sata M, 2004)
http://www.ncbi.nlm.nih.gov/sites/entrez?Db=pubmed&Cmd=ShowDetailView&TermToSearch=15359887&ordinalpos=1&itool=EntrezSystem2.PEntrez.Pubmed.Pubmed_ResultsPanel.Pubmed_RVDocSum

(15) The long-term effect of a plaque control program on tooth mortality, caries and periodontal disease in adults. Results after 30 years of maintenance. (Axelsson P, Nyström B, Lindhe J, 2004)
http://www.ncbi.nlm.nih.gov/sites/entrez?Db=pubmed&Cmd=ShowDetailView&TermToSearch=15312097&ordinalpos=7&itool=EntrezSystem2.PEntrez.Pubmed.Pubmed_ResultsPanel.Pubmed_RVDocSum

(16) Need for genetics education in U.S. dental and dental hygiene programs. (Behnke AR, Hassell TM, 2004)
http://www.ncbi.nlm.nih.gov/sites/entrez?Db=pubmed&Cmd=ShowDetailView&TermToSearch=15286103&ordinalpos=2&itool=EntrezSystem2.PEntrez.Pubmed.Pubmed_ResultsPanel.Pubmed_RVDocSum

(17) Can nonstandardized bitewing radiographs be used to assess the presence of alveolar bone loss in epidemiologic studies? (Merchant AT, Pitiphat W, Parker J, Joshipura K, Kellerman M, Douglass CW, 2004)
http://www.ncbi.nlm.nih.gov/sites/entrez

(18) Comparison of plaque removing ability of one standard and two flexible-head toothbrushes. (Warren DP, Rice HC, Turner S, 2004)
http://www.ncbi.nlm.nih.gov/sites/entrez?Db=pubmed&Cmd=ShowDetailView&TermToSearch=15190690&ordinalpos=1&itool=EntrezSystem2.PEntrez.Pubmed.Pubmed_ResultsPanel.Pubmed_RVDocSum

(19) Dental hygienists and oral cancer prevention: Knowledge, attitudes and behaviors in Italy. (Nicotera G, Gnisci F, Bianco A, Angelillo IF, 2004)
http://www.ncbi.nlm.nih.gov/sites/entrez?Db=pubmed&Cmd=ShowDetailView&TermToSearch=15063393&ordinalpos=12&itool=EntrezSystem2.PEntrez.Pubmed.Pubmed_ResultsPanel.Pubmed_RVDocSum

(20) Maximizing the dental workforce: implications for a rural state. (Krause D, Mosca N, Livingston N, 2003)
http://www.ncbi.nlm.nih.gov/sites/entrez?Db=pubmed&Cmd=ShowDetailView&TermToSearch=15022525&ordinalpos=2&itool=EntrezSystem2.PEntrez.Pubmed.Pubmed_ResultsPanel.Pubmed_RVDocSum

(21) Radiographic detection of approximal caries: a comparison between senior dental students and senior dental hygiene students. (Wojtowicz PA, Brooks SL, Hasson H, Kerschbaum WE, Eklund SA,

2003)
http://www.ncbi.nlm.nih.gov/sites/entrez?db=pubmed&cmd=search&term=radiographic%20detection%20of%20approximal%20caries:%20a%20comparison%20between%20senior%20dental%20students

(22) Quantification of dental plaque in the research environment. (Pretty IA, Edgar WM, Smith PW, Higham SM, 2005)
http://www.ncbi.nlm.nih.gov/sites/entrez?Db=pubmed&Cmd=ShowDetailView&TermToSearch=15725520&ordinalpos=11&itool=EntrezSystem2.PEntrez.Pubmed.Pubmed_ResultsPanel.Pubmed_RVDocSum

(23) Plaque and gingivitis reduction in patients undergoing orthodontic treatment with fixed appliances-compariso of toothbrushes and interdental cleaning aids a 6-month clinical single-blind trial. (Kossack C, Jost-Brinkmann PG, 2005)
http://www.ncbi.nlm.nih.gov/sites/entrez?Db=pubmed&Cmd=ShowDetailView&TermToSearch=15711898&ordinalpos=1&itool=EntrezSystem2.PEntrez.Pubmed.Pubmed_ResultsPanel.Pubmed_RVDocSum

(24) Gingival enlargement in children treated with antiepileptics. (Tan H, Gürbüz T, Da_suyu IM, 2004)
http://www.ncbi.nlm.nih.gov/sites/entrez?Db=pubmed&Cmd=ShowDetailView&TermToSearch=15704870&ordinalpos=7&itool=EntrezSystem2.PEntrez.Pubmed.Pubmed_ResultsPanel.Pubmed_RVDocSum

(25) Extrinsic tooth stain removal efficacy of a sodium bicarbonate dual-phase dentifrice containing calcium and phosphate in a six-week clinical trial. (Putt MS, Milleman JL, Ghassemi A, 2004)
http://www.ncbi.nlm.nih.gov/sites/entrez?Db=pubmed&Cmd=ShowDetailView&TermToSearch=15688962&ordinalpos=4&itool=EntrezSystem2.PEntrez.Pubmed.Pubmed_ResultsPanel.Pubmed_RVDocSum

(26) Teaching oral hygiene to children with autism. (Pilebro C, Bäckman B, 2005)
http://www.ncbi.nlm.nih.gov/sites/entrez?Db=pubmed&Cmd=ShowDetailView&TermToSearch=15663439&ordinalpos=1&itool=EntrezSystem2.PEntrez.Pubmed.Pubmed_ResultsPanel.Pubmed_RVDocSum

(27) Prioritizing oral health in pregnancy. (Breedlove G, 2004)
http://www.ncbi.nlm.nih.gov/sites/entrez

(28) Interproximal plaque mass and fluoride retention after brushing and flossing: a comparative study of powered toothbrushing, manual toothbrushing and flossing. (Sjögren K, Lundberg AB, Birkhed D, Dudgeon DJ, Johnson MR, 2004)
http://www.ncbi.nlm.nih.gov/sites/entrez

(29) Evaluation of dental flossing on a group of second grade students undertaking supervised tooth brushing. (Halla-Júnior R, Oppermann RV, 2004)
http://www.ncbi.nlm.nih.gov/sites/entrez?Db=pubmed&Cmd=ShowDetailView&TermToSearch=15646944&ordinalpos=9&itool=EntrezSystem2.PEntrez.Pubmed.Pubmed_ResultsPanel.Pubmed_RVDocSum

(30) The caries balance: the basis for caries management by risk assessment. (Featherstone JD, 2004)
http://www.ncbi.nlm.nih.gov/sites/entrez?Db=pubmed&Cmd=ShowDetailView&TermToSearch=15646583&ordinalpos=1&itool=EntrezSystem2.PEntrez.Pubmed.Pubmed_ResultsPanel.Pubmed_RVDocSum

(31) Prevention and dental health services. (Widström E, 2004)
http://www.ncbi.nlm.nih.gov/sites/entrez?Db=pubmed&Cmd=ShowDetailView&TermToSearch=15646582&ordinalpos=455&itool=EntrezSystem2.PEntrez.Pubmed.Pubmed_ResultsPanel.Pubmed_RVDocSum

(32) Why is there and should there be more

263-00488

attention paid to dental erosion? (Hefferren JJ, 2004)
http://www.ncbi.nlm.nih.gov/sites/entrez

(33) Cleaning efficacy of a manual toothbrush with tapered filaments. (Dörfer CE, von Bethlenfalvy ER, Kugel B, Pioch T, 2003)
http://www.ncbi.nlm.nih.gov/sites/entrez?Db=pubmed&Cmd=ShowDetailView&TermToSearch=15645932&ordinalpos=9&itool=EntrezSystem2.PEntrez.Pubmed.Pubmed_ResultsPanel.Pubmed_RVDocSum

(34) Comparative effect of chewing sticks and toothbrushing on plaque removal and gingival health. (Al-Otaibi M, Al-Harthy M, Söder B, Gustafsson A, Angmar-Månsson B, 2003)
http://www.ncbi.nlm.nih.gov/sites/entrez?Db=pubmed&Cmd=ShowDetailView&TermToSearch=15643758&ordinalpos=1&itool=EntrezSystem2.PEntrez.Pubmed.Pubmed_ResultsPanel.Pubmed_RVDocSum

(35) Self-reported oral health, dental care habits and cardiovascular disease in an adult Swedish population. (Buhlin K, Gustafsson A, Håkansson J, Klinge B, 2003)
http://www.ncbi.nlm.nih.gov/sites/entrez?Db=pubmed&Cmd=ShowDetailView&TermToSearch=15643757&ordinalpos=6&itool=EntrezSystem2.PEntrez.Pubmed.Pubmed_ResultsPanel.Pubmed_RVDocSum

(36) Long-term effect of an oral hygiene training program on knowledge and reported behavior. (Mayer MP, de Paiva Buischi Y, de Oliveira LB, Gjermo O, 2003)
http://www.ncbi.nlm.nih.gov/sites/entrez?Db=pubmed&Cmd=ShowDetailView&TermToSearch=15643747&ordinalpos=4&itool=EntrezSystem2.PEntrez.Pubmed.Pubmed_ResultsPanel.Pubmed_RVDocSum

(37) Periodontal risk assessment (PRA) for patients in supportive periodontal therapy (SPT). (Lang NP, Tonetti MS, 2003)
http://www.ncbi.nlm.nih.gov/sites/entrez?Db=pubmed&Cmd=ShowDetailView&TermToSearch=15643744&ordinalpos=19&itool=EntrezSystem2.PEntrez.Pubmed.Pubmed_ResultsPanel.Pubmed_RVDocSum

(38) Three different rinsing times and inhibition of plaque accumulation with chlorhexidine. (Van der Weijden GA, Timmerman MF, Novotny AG, Rosema NA, Verkerk AA, 2005)
http://www.ncbi.nlm.nih.gov/sites/entrez?Db=pubmed&Cmd=ShowDetailView&TermToSearch=15642064&ordinalpos=1&itool=EntrezSystem2.PEntrez.Pubmed.Pubmed_ResultsPanel.Pubmed_RVDocSum

(39) Relationships between lifestyle and dental health behaviors in a rural population in Japan. (Harada S, Akhter R, Kurita K, Mori M, Hoshikoshi M, Tamashiro H, Morita M, 2005)
http://www.ncbi.nlm.nih.gov/sites/entrez?Db=pubmed&Cmd=ShowDetailView&TermToSearch=15642043&ordinalpos=2&itool=EntrezSystem2.PEntrez.Pubmed.Pubmed_ResultsPanel.Pubmed_RVDocSum

(40) Lactic acid formation in supragingival dental plaque after schoolchildren's intake of fluoridated milk. (Engström K, Sjöström I, Petersson LG, Twetman S, 2004)
http://www.ncbi.nlm.nih.gov/sites/entrez?Db=pubmed&Cmd=ShowDetailView&TermToSearch=15641760&ordinalpos=1&itool=EntrezSystem2.PEntrez.Pubmed.Pubmed_ResultsPanel.Pubmed_RVDocSum

(41) The 'Significant Caries Index' (SiC): a critical approach. (Campus G, Solinas G, Maida C, Castiglia P, 2003)
http://www.ncbi.nlm.nih.gov/sites/entrez

(42) Stain reduction of an integrated oral hygiene system. (Nunn ME, Chaves ES, Gallagher AC, Rodriguez SM, Ortblad KM, 2004)
http://www.ncbi.nlm.nih.gov/sites/entrez

(43) Brushing compliance with a novel integrated power toothbrush and toothpaste oral hygiene system. (Rethman J, Neusser F, Bar AP, 2004)
http://www.ncbi.nlm.nih.gov/sites/entrez?Db=pubmed&Cmd=ShowDetailView&TermToSearch=15637978&ordinalpos=18&itool=EntrezSystem2.PEntrez.Pubmed.Pubmed_ResultsPanel.Pubmed_RVDocSum

(44) Effect of a novel integrated power toothbrush and toothpaste oral hygiene system on gingivitis. (Barlow AP, Zhou X, Roberts J, Colgan P, 2004)
http://www.ncbi.nlm.nih.gov/sites/entrez?Db=pubmed&Cmd=ShowDetailView&TermToSearch=15637976&ordinalpos=2&itool=EntrezSystem2.PEntrez.Pubmed.Pubmed_ResultsPanel.Pubmed_RVDocSum

(45) Plaque reduction over time of an integrated oral hygiene system. (Nunn ME, Ruhlman CD, Mallatt PR, Rodriguez SM, Ortblad KM, 2004)
http://www.ncbi.nlm.nih.gov/sites/entrez

(46) Team care for periodontal diseases: a model for patient rights. (Townsend C, 2004)
http://www.ncbi.nlm.nih.gov/sites/entrez?Db=pubmed&Cmd=ShowDetailView&TermToSearch=15633827&ordinalpos=1&itool=EntrezSystem2.PEntrez.Pubmed.Pubmed_ResultsPanel.Pubmed_RVDocSum

(47) Oral health in Jordan. (Taani DS, 2004)
http://www.ncbi.nlm.nih.gov/sites/entrez?Db=pubmed&Cmd=ShowDetailView&TermToSearch=15631103&ordinalpos=12&itool=EntrezSystem2.PEntrez.Pubmed.Pubmed_ResultsPanel.Pubmed_RVDocSum

(48) Classification system for toothbrushing habits. (Kujirai M, 2004)
http://www.ncbi.nlm.nih.gov/sites/entrez?Db=pubmed&Cmd=ShowDetailView&TermToSearch=15612343&ordinalpos=2&itool=EntrezSystem2.PEntrez.Pubmed.Pubmed_ResultsPanel.Pubmed_RVDocSum

(49) Fluoride gel inhibits caries in children who have low caries-risk but this may not be clinically relevant. (Marinho V, 2004)
http://www.ncbi.nlm.nih.gov/sites/entrez?Db=pubmed&Cmd=ShowDetailView&TermToSearch=15608707&ordinalpos=3&itool=EntrezSystem2.PEntrez.Pubmed.Pubmed_ResultsPanel.Pubmed_RVDocSum

(50) A practical guide to infant oral health. (Douglass JM, Douglass AB, Silk HJ, 2004)
http://www.ncbi.nlm.nih.gov/sites/entrez?Db=pubmed&Cmd=ShowDetailView&TermToSearch=15606059&ordinalpos=1&itool=EntrezSystem2.PEntrez.Pubmed.Pubmed_ResultsPanel.Pubmed_RVDocSum

3. Organization for Safety and Asepsis Procedures (OSAP)
http://www.osap.org/

4. ADA (American Dental Association), Dental Professionals
http://www.ada.org/prof/index.asp

5. The Canadian Dental Hygienists Association (CDHA)
http://www.cdha.ca/

6. The Wisdom Tooth Home Page
http://www.umanitoba.ca/outreach/wisdomtooth/

7. The American Dental Hygienists' Association (ADHA), Kids stuff
http://www.adha.org/kidstuff/index.html

8. Healthy Teeth (Oral health education database, Nova Scotia Dental Association: Healthy Teeth)
http://www.healthyteeth.org/

9. The British Society of Dental Hygiene and Therapy (BSDHT)
http://www.bdha.org.uk/

263-00488

INDEX

263-00488

263-00488

263-00488

263-00488

263-00488

263-00488

263-00488

263-00488

●す●

●せ●

●そ●

●た●

263-00488

263-00488

【著者略歴】

Thomas R. Ward（トーマス　ウォード）

1968 年　ミシガン大学卒業
1982 年　ウエストバージニア大学歯学部卒業
1983 年　日本の歯科医師免許取得
1984 年～現在　大阪歯科大学非常勤講師
1990～2012 年　東京クリニックデンタルオフィス

川口　陽子（かわぐち　ようこ）

1979 年　東京医科歯科大学歯学部卒業
　　　　東京医科歯科大学歯学部予防歯科学講座助手
1996 年　東京医科歯科大学歯学部予防歯科学講座講師
2000 年　東京医科歯科大学大学院健康推進歯学分野教授
2020 年　東京医科歯科大学名誉教授

廣瀬　浩二（ひろせ　こうじ）

1979 年　日本大学文理学部卒業
1994 年　上越教育大学大学院学校教育研究科修了
1999 年　明倫短期大学歯科衛生士学科助教授（現 准教授）
2003 年　バーミンガム大学大学院英語学科修了
2014 年　レスター大学大学院博士課程修了
　　　　EdD in Applied Linguistics and TESOL
2019 年　東京農業大学農学部外国語研究室教授

杉田めぐみ（すぎた）

1997 年　横浜国立大学大学院教育学研究科英語教育専攻修了
2000 年　ハワイ大学大学院 Department of Second
　　　　Language Studies 修了
2009 年　千葉県立保健医療大学講師
2015 年　神田外語大学外国語学部講師
2021 年　神田外語大学外国語学部准教授

【編者略歴】

矢尾　和彦（やお　かずひこ）

1965 年　大阪歯科大学卒業
1975 年　歯学博士
1991 年　大阪歯科大学助教授（小児歯科学講座）
1995～2008 年　同大学歯科衛生士専門学校校長

高阪　利美（こうさか　としみ）

1974 年　愛知学院大学歯科衛生士学院卒業
1982 年　愛知学院短期大学卒業
1993 年　愛知学院大学歯科衛生専門学校教務主任
2004 年　佛教大学社会福祉学科卒業
2006 年　愛知学院大学短期大学部歯科衛生学科准教授
2012 年　愛知学院大学短期大学部歯科衛生学科教授
2021 年　愛知学院大学特任教授

合場千佳子（あいばちかこ）

1980 年　日本歯科大学附属歯科専門学校卒業
1997 年　明星大学人文学部卒業
2006 年　立教大学異文化コミュニケーション研究科修士課程修了
2011 年　愛知学院大学大学院歯学研究科博士課程修了（歯学博士）
2012 年　日本歯科大学東京短期大学歯科衛生学科教授

263-00488

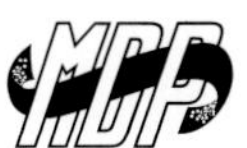

※ 本書は『最新歯科衛生士教本』の内容を引き継ぎ，必要な箇所の見直しを行ったものです．

歯科衛生学シリーズ
歯科英語　ISBN978-4-263-42620-3

2023年 1月 20日　第1版第1刷発行
2024年 1月 20日　第1版第2刷発行

監　修　一般社団法人
全国歯科衛生士
教育協議会
著　者　Thomas R. Ward ほか
発行者　白　石　泰　夫
発行所　**医歯薬出版株式会社**
〒113-8612　東京都文京区本駒込1-7-10
TEL.（03）5395-7638（編集）・7630（販売）
FAX.（03）5395-7639（編集）・7633（販売）
https://www.ishiyaku.co.jp/
郵便振替番号　00190-5-13816

乱丁，落丁の際はお取り替えいたします　印刷・第一印刷所／製本・愛千製本所